LARRY NORTH'S

SLIMDOWN FOR LIFE

D0032888

LARRY NORTH'S

SLIMDOWN FOR LIFE

LARRY NORTH

KENSINGTON BOOKS
Kensington Publishing Corp.
http://www.kensingtonbooks.com

To David Lucas, my best friend from high school, who died of a massive heart attack on the very day I finished this book. David, who was only 37, was the one who first encouraged me, when I was still a tall, overweight kid, to go into the weight room. He became my trainer and my motivator. He was twenty years ahead of his time when it came to training. He was an incredible man. He oozed with passion. He didn't believe in words like "no" or "can't." His work ethic was incomparable to anyone I have ever met in my life. And incredibly, he always believed in me. David, I love you. Your heart failed prematurely, but you will always be in my heart.

Your longtime high school pal,

Larry North

For information about Slim Down products,
call
1-800-371-9264.

If you are interested in finding out the latest
news about health and fitness, be sure to
sign on to my Web site at:

http://www.larrynorth.com/

Acknowledgments

It is always so difficult for me to write acknowledgments because I personally feel that the only people who read them are the ones I mentioned or those I inadvertently forgot to mention. The reality is that there have been so many people who have had a profound influence on me. I have so many people to thank for helping me reach this point of my life.

My wife, Melanie Peskett North, created all of the wonderful recipes in this book. She is a wonderful chef, and she prepares these recipes for me at home. She brings incredible happiness into my life.

To my mother, Beverly Miller-North, and my brothers, Adam and Alan—my love for you, and the love we have for each other, is the most powerful influence in our universe.

Many accolades to my editor, Paul Dinas; my literary agent, David Hale Smith of DHS Literary (along with his associates Seth Robertson and Shelley Lewis); my agent/manager, Verna Riddles; all the fine people at Larry North Fitness, Larry North Sports Medicine, Larry North *Health and Fitness Insider, Good Morning Texas* television show, and radio station KRLD. Also, a very special thank-you to Kensington Publishing.

There are not enough words to express my appreciation to Keith Klein. To me, he is the finest nutritionist on the planet, and he has been greatly influential in educating me about fitness and nutrition. Also, heartfelt thanks to Joey Antonio and Chris Street for their scientific editing. Thanks to Skip Hollandsworth for his writing advice. You are all experts in your fields and have greatly assisted me in sending the right message to the public.

I would especially like to thank fitness expert Everett Aaberg for his technical advice and literary contribution to the exercise portion of this book. Utilizing his expertise of biomechanics and his extensive knowledge of the design and function of the human body ensures that the exercises and stretches in this book will be of maximum benefit with minimal risk to all of you performing them. He is definitely one of the top instructors, personal trainers, and authors on fitness in the country.

I am very proud to call Darwin Deason my dear friend and early-morning workout partner. Darwin, I'll see you in the gym at 5:30 (that's A.M.!).

I want to express my appreciation to the entire gang at the No. 1 infomercial company, Quantum Television, especially Jack Kirby, Brady Caverly, John Boyle, and Andy Spivak for developing *The Great North American Slimdown* and making it the No. 1 infomercial for 1998.

There are many more individuals who are special to me: Cathy Odom, my assistant and friend, Skip Bayless, Joe Mauro, Doug Murphy, and Chris Gallagher. God bless. I love you all.

And finally, to my very important audience, I dedicate this book to you. I feel that *Larry North's Slimdown for Life* will be the final book you will ever need about eating and exercise.

Contents

A Real Program for Real People

Finally, Your Opportunity to Get the Body You Want

Any program that you can't do for the rest of your life is not worth doing for a single day.

This is going to be the simplest book about food and fitness that you will ever read.

I mean, really simple.

You're not going to learn anything about food pyramids. You won't need calorie-counting charts. You're not going have to walk around a grocery store with a calculator figuring out fat grams. And you're not going to have to order any of those absurdly complicated contraptions that are advertised on informercials which promise you the perfect body.

And most important, you're not going to read one word about "dieting." Not one. I'm not into fads. I'm not into myths. And I have made it my mission in life to destroy the myths that have held so many of you back for far too long.

I'll bet many of you still believe you must radically cut back on food and starve yourself in order to get thin.

I'll show you exactly the opposite is true.

Many of you have heard the myth that says the best way for you to burn the excess fat off your body is through some exhausting, superintense aerobics and weight-lifting workout.

Again not true.

If you still believe you can only win the weight game by constantly depriving your body of healthful food— i.e., dieting—and if you still believe that the way to get a great body is to work out until you drop, then you have missed the revolution that can completely change your life.

Well, now the time has come.

Here is the very simple truth: The only way to get lean—and to stay lean permanently—is through regular low-fat eating and through very moderate exercise. I know such words as "moderation," "balance," and "steadiness" sound boring. But those are the words that work—as long as you find a program that can integrate those habits into your own life.

And that's where this book—*Larry North's Slimdown for Life*—comes in. For years, I have been working to develop exactly the program that doesn't require you to change your lifestyle but enhances your lifestyle. It's a program that doesn't force you to overhaul your life, but one that leads you to embrace the kind of positive habits that will start transforming your body.

This is the program for the millions of people out there who have not been doing a thing to get a better body, in large part because they are so confused from the vast amounts of misinformation being thrown at them. This is the program for those of you who are desperate to lose weight, but who never seem to get started on a weight-loss program because you're too intimidated by all the exercise routines and dieting that you *think* you have to do.

Are you ready to join the revolution? To join the hundreds of thousands of Americans who are using this program right now to change their bodies, their attitudes, and their lives?

Discovering the Slimdown for Life

Let me tell you about who I am and how I came to develop the Slimdown for Life program. I grew up in a world where everyone in my family fought a losing battle with weight. My grandmother weighed nearly 300 pounds. When my mother was six years old, she was already the fattest girl in the neighborhood. Every night, after suffering through countless insults from other kids, she cried herself to sleep. By the time she was eleven, she was already going to a diet doctor. He prescribed diet pills and gave her two boxes of appetite-suppressant chocolate candy—both boxes of which she ate on the way home. And that was just the beginning. My mom, who joined the very first Overeaters Anonymous chapter in the country, spent the rest of her life obsessed about losing weight. She would try to starve herself all week, then take her diet pills (which were, of course, amphetamines) and then find herself bingeing through the weekend.

There were times when I couldn't believe what I was seeing. My mom got so addicted to those diet pills that she needed them not to lose weight but just to stay awake through the day. She went for weeks eating nothing but hard-boiled eggs and cottage cheese. She tried diuretics and every laxative on the shelf. After reading in a magazine that pineapples were the way to lose weight, she ate so many pineapples that she went around with her lips puckered. After reading another story that fat from meat could seep through her pores, she started wearing rubber gloves when preparing food.

When people ask me why I got into the business of teaching others how to lose weight, I tell them about one afternoon when I was out with my mother. I was eleven years old, and I bought a hot dog, using my carefully hoarded allowance money. A woman relative, then on one of her 500-calorie-a-day diets, suddenly shouted, "Look over there, Larry, there's your father!" As I turned around, she grabbed my hot dog and stuck the whole thing in her mouth! I started to cry. It was a painful lesson for us both—how obsessive dieting can make you desperate.

By the time I left high school, I was determined to make my living in the fitness and weight loss business. After several years, I did develop a national reputation as a fitness guru. I wrote two highly praised books on creating the perfect body. I became a specialist at helping others become bodybuilders.

Because of my reputation as a motivator, I spoke all over the world, even as far away as New Zealand to a conference of prominent international chief executives, about the joys of reshaping one's body. I appeared on dozens of talk shows, including CNN's *Larry King Live,* exhorting America to strip away its fat. I built several gyms around Dallas and Fort Worth, which became packed with more than 30,000 members. I had a weekly syndicated radio show on fitness in which I'd go on and on about the joys of doing sit-ups and bench presses and eating tuna out of a can.

But as time passed, I realized I was not reaching the audience I wanted to reach—people like my own mother. Indeed, I kept coming across reports that showed Americans were fatter than ever before—and getting even fatter! In 1996, for example, a federal government survey found that more than 60 million people in the United States weighed 20 percent more than their ideal weight—making them, in cold medical terms, obese. In the summer of 1998, the National Institutes of Health reevaluated that report and decided that actually *97 million* Americans were "overweight." Some experts feel that the number will double by the year 2020.

So I decided to change. I started orienting my radio show to people who were fed up with the claims of cheap weight-loss programs and annoyed with fat farms and liquid formulas. They were frustrated and depressed, tired and run-down, their self-confidence shattered because they could not seem to keep the weight off. Maybe you're one of them.

I will never forget the day when I told my listeners that I wanted to hear only from those who felt absolutely hopeless about getting lean. Within minutes, a woman called and in a hesitant voice said, "Larry, all my life I've been called a success. I'm in my early forties, I'm in a high-paying profession, I'm a good mother, a good wife . . ."

Then her voice faltered. "But no matter what I've done, there is one thing I live with every day. I feel sick walking out the door of my house because of my body. I've tried everything. I've done diets, I've taken diet pills, I've gone two hours straight on a treadmill. And

I'm still over a hundred and fifty pounds. Is there anything you can do for someone like me?"

A couple of minutes later, a forty-year-old lawyer called. He told me he had put on fifty pounds over the past ten years, most of it around his midsection. He told me he had tried five different diets in the past year. Quietly, I asked him how he felt. "Larry," he said, "I didn't know I could feel so unhappy."

I listened to people who seemed so shattered. There was a woman who told me she was trying to eat just one meal a day, a man who told me he was eating only snacks, a woman who said she was eating a combination of cottage cheese and Caesar salads, another woman who said she was eating all fattening foods the first thing in the morning and then trying to eat only lettuce in the afternoon and fruit juice at night. Some guy told me that he believed he could eat anything he wanted because he worked out two hours a day. Another guy said he knew he wasn't eating fattening foods because he was tearing the skin off fried chicken. One woman thought she was going to lose weight because she ate a lot of foods that claimed to be nonfat.

As the days went on, I listened to callers talk about what it was like to try to sit through meals barely eating, to do aerobics for hours until their knees were swollen to the size of softballs, to stare at themselves in the mirror and wonder, "Why? Why does nothing change?" I remember a woman weeping during a conversation as she told me that she got so hungry late at night during her diets that she believed she was going insane. During a show one afternoon I just stared at the console in the radio booth, looking at the blinking lights signaling more calls. All the phones were lighting up. "My God," I thought, "it's an epidemic. No one knows what to do.

People are subjecting themselves to lives of dieting or exercising hell, and it's not working.''

Get Ready to Go North!

So I vowed to create a program that naturally and painlessly could be incorporated into someone's life— a program for those who didn't have time to spend hours working out, those who were too busy struggling to meet their house payments or keep their kids fed, those who felt so overweight that they were just too embarrassed to do any exercise at all. It would be a program that would appeal to overstressed executives and overworked housewives, those who were trying to handle two jobs along with those trying to handle two children.

After much study and research, after a lot of fine-tuning and tinkering, I first introduced this program in 1997 through a television infomercial—an infomercial that, incidentally, had no gizmos, no bells or whistles, and no goofy pieces of equipment allegedly designed to give you firmer abs or a tighter butt. It was just me talking about the joyful simplicity of getting rid of your fat and reshaping your body. The response was astonishing. The infomercial sold nearly half a million units through the fall of 1998 and became the best-selling weight-loss infomercial on television. I received hundreds of letters and calls from people thanking me for giving them a clear path to follow the rest of their lives. I received letters from viewers who had lost more than fifty pounds. Even though I had insisted that this was not a program designed for wannabe bodybuilders or bathing beauty babes, it turned out that a mother of three children who never had time to join a gym got on the Slimdown for Life, lost several dozen pounds, and ended up winning the title of Mrs. Plano in suburban Dallas. I was on the streets of New York City one afternoon and a construction worker yelled at me from across the street in his big Bronx accent, "Hey, Larry North, I'm doing your program and I've lost fifteen pounds!"

With this book, you are getting my program in exact detail. It is laid out in such a way that you will never be at a loss about what to do. It will guide you, almost hour by hour, for the next twenty-one days. It is remarkably easy to understand, simple to follow, and leads to lasting results.

It's also a program designed so that you think I am there with you every day, acting as your own personal trainer, someone who will shoot straight with you and tell you exactly what you need to be doing. I'll be there not only to educate you but to inspire you and, I hope, to entertain you. I will leave nothing to chance. If you want to lose weight, all you have to do is follow this step-by-step, meal-by-meal, day-by-day guide to your life for the next three weeks. You will have a specific script that will produce maximum, healthy results and rev up your metabolism, which, as you'll later learn, is a critical but often-ignored element in weight loss. In the end, you'll realize that you are getting great results—scientifically verifiable results. If you follow the program, there is no way you will fail to eliminate fat and see wonderful changes to your body. The only way not to succeed is not to try.

The Key Is Simplicity

I have made sure that the Slimdown for Life is the essence of the gentle, moderate program. Why? To sell more books? Of course not. It's because it's only through moderation that you permanently change the way you look. Rather than forcing you to starve yourself as if you were a prisoner in a concentration camp, the Slimdown for Life literally has you eating plenty of healthful, tasty foods to get a better body, using frequent meals with specific food combinations that actually burn off fat. Rather than forcing you to beat the excess calories out of your body with wildly punishing or complicated workout routines, this program has you taking a small amount of time for unstressful but still very effective exercise, focusing on a simple walking program and mild muscle-building workouts, called Sixty-Second Workouts, which last no more than a minute.

Every day, you'll progress with an eating program that gradually eliminates the foods that contain higher fat and replaces them with foods rich in proteins and complex carbohydrates (I call them starchy carbs). Every day, you'll do little exercises that start bringing back the sexier contours of your body. And every day, you'll work on your attitude—because if you are not feeling great about yourself and optimistic about what you're doing, you won't stay with this or any other program. Instead of focusing on your "willpower," as you have in the past to try to stay committed to a crazy, self-destructive diet, you'll focus on your "goal power" so that you can relish the benefits of slow, steady progress—the only kind of progress that counts when it comes to weight loss.

I remember several years ago receiving a long-distance phone call from my younger brother Alan, who told me that he was in great shape. So I invited him to move to Dallas to help run my new gym. When Alan stepped off the plane, I was speechless. What could I say? He was close to 300 pounds. He was just like everyone else in our family, prone to getting heavy at the drop of a hat. He was near tears when he looked at me. He told me that he had lied to me because he was afraid of what I would say if I knew the truth. He told me he had tried everything the rest of us had tried—and yet he kept getting heavier and heavier.

My heart broke for my brother. And at that moment, I said to myself that if I couldn't help my own brother become successful with his weight problem, then I didn't have a right to help anyone else. I took him to lunch and I said, "Get ready." I ordered him a grilled chicken breast, a serving of rice, and a salad with no-fat dressing. "Eat this, and in three hours we'll eat again," I said.

Alan stared at me. "Larry, how am I going to lose weight eating all this food?"

"Alan, this is the program. You're going to be eating these kinds of meals all the time. You're going to do some cardio work and some very light resistance exercise. You're going to learn to feed your muscle and starve your fat."

He looked at me. "What?" he said. "I'm going to what?"

I smiled. "Trust me, Alan."

I made him a trainer, put him to work in my gym, and told him his first client would be an accountant named Gary, who literally weighed 445 pounds. The first time Gary came into the gym, he could barely fit through the door. I was terrified what would happen whenever he sat down on one of my chairs. (At that point, I was just getting started in my business and didn't have many chairs.) At his first workout, Gary walked for five minutes on a treadmill at the lowest speed possible. He was so out of breath that he could barely take another step. He couldn't do any weight machines because he couldn't fit in them.

To almost everyone else in the gym, Gary and Alan seemed destined for failure. Their situations appeared hopeless. Like Alan, Gary had gone through dozens of diets and kept thinking his failures were all about a lack of "willpower."

But the two of them promised they would follow my rules, even if the rules didn't seem to make sense. They started eating five low-fat meals a day. They learned to special order in restaurants to get rid of the excess fat— just as you're going to learn to do. They learned to make good food decisions in places like movie theaters, convenience stores, and even at friends' homes to keep the fat out of their bodies. They learned to pre-prepare easy and healthful low-fat meals at home, just as you will. And they began to gently incorporate exercise into their lives, refusing to exert themselves too much—just as you will, too.

And they learned to do it anywhere they were. Gary, who traveled a lot, began a walking program, walking around the parking lots of hotels if he had to. He realized that he could walk anywhere. He never had to miss a walking workout. He also learned he could do his Sixty-Second Workouts in his hotel room or his office. Within eight weeks, he was doing ten minutes' worth of Sixty-Second Workouts and walking forty-five minutes a day. A few weeks later, he was walking at such a fast sixty-minute pace that his own twenty-year-old daughter couldn't keep up with him.

By using the very same program that you are about to do, doing nothing more or nothing less, Gary's body changed radically. In his first seven months, he lost 190 pounds. As more months passed, he lost 34 inches off his waist and went down to 218 pounds. Meanwhile, Alan went through his own remarkable changes. In four months, he dropped 100 pounds and became one of the most popular and knowledgeable trainers in the gym.

The story of Gary and Alan is not one of those cheap before-and-after stories you read in magazine ads. This is the real thing. No diet, no three-day-a-week workouts in the weight room, no medically supervised fasting. All you have to do is read this book, one day at a time. You don't have to look up the number of calories for anything you eat. You don't have to weigh food. You don't have to learn some system of "food exchanges." You just have to relax and do what I tell you and get ready to lose weight forever.

Your Own Personal Trainer

So once again, let me ask you, "Are you ready to join the revolution?" All I'm asking for are three weeks of your life. I'll be there with you the first thing in the morning, and I'll be there at the very end of the day to talk about what we've accomplished. In between, I'll give you small minilectures on food and fitness. I'll explain why certain exercises work for you and why certain foods can sabotage your weight. Each day, I'll pause and answer the questions that naturally start arising as you go through the program, and in the process, I'll knock down all the mind-boggling junk that other so-called experts have tried to pass off as fact. And I'll be giving you so many pep talks to keep you motivated that you'll want to run through a wall.

For each day, I'll give you suggestions on exactly what to eat at each meal and which workouts to do. You'll learn in detail how to follow a simple but powerful walking program that lets you progress at your own pace, and to make sure you do the Sixty-Second Workouts correctly, I've provided photographs and detailed instructions to twenty-two routines, from leg raises in a chair to modified push-ups off a table. You'll never again feel that you don't have time to work out, for these are exercises you will be able to do when you're sitting at the office or watching a ballgame or playing with your children.

I also have devoted a chapter in the back of the book entirely to recipes. If you have leafed through other low-fat cookbooks, then your head probably starts spinning as mine does at the sight of all the complicated recipes. But these recipes are so astonishingly easy, they take little time in the kitchen. They reproduce many of your favorite foods—only they are all very low fat. Just look at the recipes for Cheese Grits or Seven-Layer Dip, the Taco Salad or Strawberry Cheesecake Dream. This is not the kind of food that you eat and think, "Well, at least I'm doing something healthy for myself." Hey, I love good food—and I have made absolutely sure the food you get in this program is absolutely great, too.

You'll also get a detailed eating-out guide that will show you little things to do at restaurants that will cut out huge amounts of fat from your food. You'll learn how to "special order" when you eat out, and you'll learn to make better choices if you decide to have a higher-fat meal or snack. And finally, as an extra benefit for you after your completion of the 21-day program, I have added a special miniprogram that I call the *Seven-Day Sizedown*. If you are facing an upcoming wedding or party or class reunion or trip to the beach, and you want to get as lean as possible, the Seven-Day Sizedown is a brief but very intense one-week routine to strip out the fat from your diet and push you to burn off far more calories than usual through extra workouts. Some of you won't ever need it—and trust me, it's not the kind of program on which to base the rest of your life. But if you need something in a pinch, this is it.

Remember, there are no rules, only suggestions. The more suggestions you adopt, the faster you'll see results.

I'm not sure there is any other place where you can find such an amazing variety of information about health and fitness, set up so that you can easily integrate it all into your life over the next twenty-one days. I'm giving you everything I know—every trick I've discovered to outwit your fat cells, every technique to build your muscle tissue, every method I have to stay motivated and emotionally pumped up. You will not be able to read any page of this book without thinking, "I can do this! I can do this!"

So take a deep breath and put aside every notion you ever had about diets. You are about to head off on a new road to healthiness, wholeness, and fitness. You have the chance to bring back the contours in your body, to knock off the weight from your hips and thighs. Just imagine a day in which the idea of food does not bring up any negative or guilty thoughts inside you. Imagine a day where you actually can enjoy sitting down to eat, because you know you are leading a healthy life, because you know that you control food rather than it controlling you. Imagine a day in which your feelings about your body are so positive that your whole life is transformed. Imagine eliminating all the psychological burden that has built up in your life due to your deep anxiety about food and weight.

Can you really imagine it? Well, listen to me. The

time has come to believe in that freedom. That life is here for you right now. All you have to do is be patient, follow me for the next twenty-one days, and trust your body to take over.

Trust the program. Trust it. You are about to get results that you simply—and I mean simply—will not believe.

Part One

The Secrets of
the Slimdown

Getting Ready to Reshape
Your Body Forever

It's not the person who diets and trains the hardest who finds success. It's the one who eats and works out the smartest.

CHAPTER

1

Know How Your Body Works

I want you to take a moment and visualize what happens when food enters your body. I am convinced that if you can picture this process, you're going to have such a different appreciation of your body—and how you can get it to work to your advantage—that you'll realize once and for all that the time has come to develop a whole new mind-set about food and fitness.

Here's what happens when you eat food. Some of the calories immediately enter the bloodstream to be used for energy. The rest go either to your lean muscle tissue, where they are burned up as fuel, or they go to your fat cells. In order to lose weight, you must confront your fat cells—and let me tell you right now, these things are remarkable adversaries.

It's the fat cells that make you look fat, and there

are 30 billion of them—that's right, *30 billion*—inside you. Altogether, they can store up to 150 pounds of fat in the average body. They have an ingenious ability to withstand most attacks we throw at them. You cannot starve these fat cells out of existence. You cannot get rid of them by running twenty miles a week. They are there forever, just underneath your skin, in your blood, your muscles and organs with one purpose only: to store calories. They don't like to give up their calories under any circumstances.

And your fat cells will turn into vicious beasts when you start restricting the number of calories entering your body.

Do you think I'm exaggerating? To get an understanding of how powerful our fat cells can be, you have to go back thousands of years, to periods in history when human beings went through genuine famines and droughts. We are descendants of people whose bodies were able to survive the kinds of food shortages from ancient times that could lead to mass starvation. Those who didn't die during those famines were those people who possessed—you guessed it—enough body fat. Their bodies were able to efficiently store enough calories in their fat cells to survive the famines. That trait was then passed on to the next generation, and to the next generation—and now to us. *In other words, you have been given a body that just loves to store fat.*

Throughout most of our lives, we have lived with the myth that the way to combat our fat cells is to just starve our bodies entirely by severely restricting our food intake. I am sure you have heard one of these best-selling dietitians from the people I call the "Diet Mafia" say that the way to lose weight is simply to cut back more calories. They grandly say that if you just cut back 500 calories a day, you're going to lose 3,500 calories at the end of the week—which is equivalent to one pound. You do that five weeks in a row? Presto. You've dropped five pounds.

Sorry. Scientists now know it doesn't work that way at all, and there is one reason why it doesn't. It's because of our fat cells. Regardless of how much willpower you think you have, your fat cells are always going to be stronger. It is a medical certainty that they will bust up any "diet" you throw at them.

"But wait, Larry," you might be saying, "whenever I have restricted my caloric intake in the past, I have lost weight."

Yes, I agree, you probably did lose weight. So let me ask you a question: Why are you reading this book?

You know the reason, don't you? It's because the weight came back, didn't it?

Granted, you will lose some weight when you cut back calories—*for a while.* Some of you will lose ten pounds in a couple of weeks, then another ten pounds in the next two weeks. Some of you will have to be able to fight your gnawing hunger for much longer. You will think, "Aha! I'm a success! I've done it!"

But during that very period of time, your body will be changing. Because of your ancient past, your fat cells are interpreting your "diet" as nothing more than a famine. As soon as these fat cells think a famine is under way, they go into crisis mode and start storing most of the calories you ingest. Have you ever wondered why you've lost some weight in the first few weeks of a diet, but then you suddenly don't lose as quickly even though you are eating the same amount? It's because your fat cells have taken on a new role in your body. It's as if they have doors that open up to get every calorie that passes by.

You can cut back on your food intake even more,

but the fat cells will keep adjusting in order to store more and more calories. And once those calories are in there, your fat cells are very reluctant to let them go.

But that's not all! I've got more bad news. To make sure that the calories stay untouched in those fat cells, the body starts looking for other sources of energy. And it invariably turns to lean muscle tissue that covers your body. This is your most metabolically active tissue, the best place to burn off calories, the very component of your body you should do everything to keep. Some studies say that up to 50 percent of the weight you lose on a standard diet can come from your muscle.

By making your muscle cells smaller and weaker, you might think you're getting thinner. But you're actually making yourself listless, less healthy, and most surprising of all, "fatter" on the inside. Instead of weighing 120 pounds with 25 percent body fat, for example, a diet has dropped you to 110 pounds but given you 30 percent body fat. And that makes things even worse for you. Because you now have less muscle in proportion to your fat, you have a greater likelihood to send more calories in the future to your fat cells.

Don't forget, your fat cell doors are wide open during a diet. And when you start eating normally again, your fat cells are ready to balloon. Mark my words, you will eat more than you can imagine because your fat cells will be sending louder and more frantic hunger signals to your brain. Eventually, those signals will get so powerful that you will want to break into Fort Knox if there's a candy bar in there. Ultimately, you'll be gaining back weight so fast that you'll probably find yourself heavier than when you started your diet in the first place.

When you undereat, you end up overeating all the foods you tried to avoid in the first place.

It's distressing, isn't it? With each diet, you are only

setting up your body to get fatter and fatter. Ask yourself: Was that your intention, to get your body to hoard calories instead of burning them?

More than 90 percent of us quit our diets after only a month—90 percent! Yet amazingly, when you decide after failing one diet to try to lose weight again, you inevitably turn once more to a . . . *diet*! You turn to the very thing that eventually will make you heavier.

Ask yourself: How crazy is that? If you ask me, the time has come to get off that merry-go-round and devise a new weight-loss strategy.

The North Secret to Slimming Down for Life

If you want to get lean, then the first thing you need to do is get the food you eat past your fat cells and into your muscle tissue, where it is easier to burn off. You want to reduce your fat cells while maintaining and even increasing your muscle cells.

And here is where the Slimdown for Life makes its entrance.

In my program, there is one great answer to lasting weight loss, and it's all about eating. Food becomes our ally. Indeed, by the end of these twenty-one days, you're going to eat every three or four hours like clockwork. You're not going to undereat at any meal, and you're not going to overeat at any meal. Most important, you're going to be eating more foods than you ever thought possible and enjoying your meals more as well.

Did you read that previous paragraph corrrectly? You did. We now have the research that proves that we do ourselves more harm than good by not eating. The same research is showing us how we can make our bodies work to our advantage through some basic changes in what we eat and how we eat, and by adding in only small amounts of exercise.

To me, this is a very exciting time. And what I've set out to do in the Slimdown for Life is to teach you how to use real food, and lots of it, to make you thinner. As strange as it sounds, you will eat to lose.

The Great Calorie Hoax

I know you're thinking, "Uh, big deal, Larry, we all know to cut back on fat." But do you really? It is amazing how few of you grasp the concept of what fat does or how much we really consume. You still do not understand that the fat that is in your food—dietary fat, it's called—has a makeup that is already very similar to that of the fat found in your body. That means your body has to do very little to turn dietary fat into body fat. Thus, fatty foods are uniquely fattening.

I know I told you at the very start of this book that you will not have to count calories as part of this program. But I do want you to understand the nature of calories so that you'll know why you must eat certain foods and try to avoid others. Everything you eat contains calories. A "calorie" is a measure of heat that fuels your body and makes it run, but don't worry about trying to understand that. All that's important for you to know is what these calories will do to you.

So many of you remain stuck on the old myth that all calories are the same, regardless of whether they come from a candy bar or from spinach. Well, that's theoretically correct—as long as those calories stay in a test tube. But when those calories get in your body, they act differently. One researcher says if you eat a piece of food that contains 200 calories that come from

the fatty part of that food, only 6 of those calories—
they are called "fat calories"—will be burned off as that
piece of food works its way through the digestive system.
The remaining 97 percent of those calories—194 calories!—head to your fat cells to add padding to your
body.

Are you starting to get the picture? All you have to
do is start eliminating fat from your diet and your body
changes. When you eat food loaded with proteins and
starchy carbs, your body not only wants to send those
foods to your muscle tissue, but has to burn a lot of
calories to break those foods down as they work their
way through the digestive system. In other words, your
body burns more calories simply because you are eating
the right foods. For instance, when you eat a piece of
food that contains 200 calories of carbohydrates, your
body has to expend close to 50 calories just to break
down those carboydrates. That's opposed to the 6 calories to deal with 200 calories of fat.

Hey, don't just take my word for it. Researchers at
Cornell University once placed a group of women on
a high-fat diet (with 35 to 40 percent of calories from
fat) and another group of women on a reduced-fat diet
(with 20 to 25 percent of their calories coming from
fat). The interesting thing about this study was that
neither group of women was asked to limit the number
of calories consumed during the day. They could pig
out! They could eat as much as they wanted. But here's
what happened. After eleven weeks, the doctors found
that while on the reduced-fat diet, the women lost twice
as much weight as they did when eating the high-fat
diet. And did you notice? There was no dieting involved
whatsoever!

Yes, your body requires some fat. Fat helps supply
the essential fatty acids, which provide a layer of protec-
tion for the body, and serve as one of the lubricators

for your joints. But how much fat do you need? Don't be misled by so-called experts who say you need to eat more fat to lose weight. You never need to add fat to your diet to get the fat your body needs. Studies show that one tablespoon of corn oil rich in linoleic acid provides all the essential fat needed by most human beings. Believe me, that amount of fat is already there in the best food. There's fat in oatmeal, and there's fat in the leanest skinned piece of chicken.

Meanwhile, we're shoveling in more excess fat than at any time in history. We are selling more potato chips, more fatty meats, and more fried fast food than ever before. There are more steak houses in this country, per capita, than at any time in our history. Studies show that the average American—that means you—gets 40 percent of his or her total calories from fat.

Bypassing Your Fat Cells

Clearly, if I could just get you to cut back some of your fat intake, the Slimdown for Life would be a success. You'd lose weight. But the great thing about this program is that you start utilizing high-quality food that is *ten times* more likely to be stored in the muscle and used as a fuel source.

There are three types of food—protein, starchy carbs, and fibrous vegetables—that will race for your muscles like thoroughbred horses.

Let me explain these three food groups in more detail:

1. *Proteins:* You want protein because it provides the amino acids necessary to make your lean muscle tissue thrive. If your body does not get enough protein in your

diet, it will start eating away at the muscles. Therefore, a diet without sufficient protein will only defeat your fat-to-muscle balance in the end.

Proteins include all your meats. Of course, some meats contain far less fat, which is what we'll push in the Slimdown for Life. These include cuts of boneless, skinless turkey breast, white-meat chicken, white fishes, egg whites, lean venison and other game meats, the very leanest cuts of beef, such as sirloin and eye of round steak, center-cut pork tenderloin, canned tuna, chicken, or turkey in water, nonfat dairy products, and protein powders.

2. *Starchy Carbs:* These provide the basic energy for your body. Carbs are the most efficiently burned foods you can take in. One warning: All carbohydrates are not alike. Simple carbohydrates comprise the kinds of food with lots of sugar and refined flour that can ruin your program, such as cakes and cookies. Simple carbohydrates that are known as "processed food"—that's just about anything that comes in a box, such as pasta and cereals—can hurt your program if you rely too much on them. We will focus on such starch carbs as brown rice, yams, grits, white potatoes, sweet potatoes, oatmeal, oat bran, corn, whole-grain breads, whole-grain pastas, shredded wheat, cream of rice, black-eyed peas, lima beans, black beans, white beans, pinto beans, and many more.

3. *Fibrous Vegetables:* Fibrous vegetables are composed primarily of water and nutrients. These include broccoli, cauliflower, carrots, green and red peppers, asparagus, celery, spinach, lettuces, green peas, tomatoes, egg-plant, green beans, squash, cabbage, radishes, onions, zucchini, and cucumbers. These foods are full of vitamins and they are invaluable to your digestive system, acting as a kind of scrubbing brush that cleans out cells

and eliminates water retention. For someone trying to lose weight, there's a special benefit to fibrous vegetables. They have very few calories, practically no fat, and because they are digested more slowly, they help you feel full more quickly. Foods with lots of fiber tend to require more chewing, so they make you eat more slowly. They also reduce the levels of insulin in your blood, a hormone that can stimulate the appetite.

Jumpstarting Your Metabolism

Here's the only scientific word you'll have to learn in this entire book: "metabolism." But it's a word that you must keep at the forefront of your brain for the next twenty-one days. Think of your metabolism as your body's inner engine. It's what keeps all the different parts of the body operating, from the beating of your heart to the blinking of your eyelids. Your metabolism— and this is very important—is also what burns most of the calories that are in the food you eat.

Some studies suggest that you burn off 75 percent of your total calories if you have a normal metabolism. But you also have the power to either speed up or slow down your metabolism. When you go on a strict diet, for example, you automatically start slowing down your metabolism whether you know it or not. Indeed, in a strict diet, your metabolism can slow to a barely perceptible crawl—which is exactly what our ancestors' bodies did during a famine in order to survive. Your body will shift into such a deep conservation mode that you will have to start cutting even more calories to keep losing weight. Yet it is a losing battle. The fewer calories you take in, the lower your metabolism drops.

But if you start eating the proteins, starchy carbs, and

fibrous vegetables that I just mentioned, and if you eat them at regular times during the day, your body's metabolic rate will rise in order to process those foods. Because those foods start burning while you eat them, they produce the kind of heat in your body that causes the metabolism to soar. In a sense, they will trigger a chain reaction that makes you burn even more calories. It's the most effective way of eating to achieve long-term success.

A Little Exercise Goes a Long Way

Finally, we attack the fat that's already in your body. And there's a way to do it: exercise. Furthermore, research has made some startling discoveries about what kind of exercise is really necessary to boost your metabolism so that you lose more weight: *gentle exercise.*

If you haven't exercised for years, don't worry. The noted *Journal of the American Medical Association* recently reported that men who get their "aerobic" exercise simply by doing everyday activities, such as walking, gardening, and engaging in light, leisure-time sports, have hearts as healthy as men who are exercising three times as much in more traditional ways. The distinguished Cooper Institute of Aerobics Research, the Dallas organization that invented the word "aerobics," no longer says that it's intense, vigorous exercise that leads to fitter bodies. The institute's exercise physiologist, Dr. John Duncan, explains, "We now know that metabolic changes occur at very moderate exercise intensities."

Did you hear that phrase? "Metabolic changes"? That's right, you can speed up your valuable metabolism by doing something other than running, other than grunting and groaning, other than leaping around like Michael Jordan.

Although we will spend most of our time in the Slim-down for Life learning to eat right, you'll also learn how to incorporate fitness into your life. It's the kind of exercise program that adds just the right charge to your body. It will give you an extra "kick" to boost the bene-fits of your eating program.

Are you wondering how you can burn enough calo-ries to lose fat by walking around the block? No doubt you've seen those charts in other books that tell you that doing a triathlon or going cross-country skiing burns a zillion more calories than walking. And of course, you've noticed those great, muscular bodies of professional athletes and said to yourself, "I've got to work out like that athlete if I want to look like him or her."

But the goal in this program is not to become a professional athlete—nor is the goal to exercise the way you did when you were sixteen years old. *Your goal is to get the physiology of your body to change so that it turns into a far better fat-burning machine.* You will do it with Sixty-Second Workouts, with mild resistance exercise, and with a walking "cardio" program. (I have a personal hatred of the word "aerobics" because it makes people think of those dreadfully difficult, knee-jarring aerobics classes.)

You'll probably think what I'm giving you is so moder-ate that I must be holding something back from you. But just stay with me. Let me show you how it all works once the 21-day program begins. Trust me: If you want to strip a layer of fat off your body, you're about to see astonishing results—all because you, ironically, *took it easy.*

CHAPTER

2

Getting Your House in Order

Your Final Preparations Before You Get Started

There is no one single great thing you must start doing in order to get lean. It's a combination of many little things.

Before our twenty-one days begin, there are a few final things you need to know. Consider this your warm-up chapter, the chapter that will get you focused, get your goals in order, and get the environment around you ready so that you will be able to take those very small, consistent steps in your daily life that will lead to remarkable changes. In this chapter, we're not only going to do a spiritual cleaning of our attitudes. We're also going to do a literal cleaning out of our kitchens.

Before you panic, I am not going to ask you to throw away everything in your pantry and refrigerator. I know other "diet" books ask you to do that, and I also know you never do it.

What I want you to do, however, is start being aware of the food that you could bring into your home that is nutritious and tasty and can go a long way in knocking fat out of your diet. Moreover, there are certain foods that can sabotage the Slimdown for Life if you rely too heavily on them. You do not need me to tell you that there are some foods in your kitchen that are difficult for you to stop eating once you get your hands on them. These are called "trigger" foods. For me, it's peanut butter, which is loaded with fat. Once I open a jar of peanut butter, I want to grab a spoon and go after it until there is no more peanut butter left.

I will never order you to eliminate any food. I believe there is a way to work the program and still get the chance to "cheat" and occasionally eat wonderfully decadent meals. But you also have to recognize that some foods are out there with your name on them. They are the goodies that can cause you to lose control and go on an eating rampage, especially if you've had a long, stressful day. As committed as I am to eating low-fat on this program, there are days when I could empty a jar of peanut butter if one was around. If I did, I would consume at least 1,000 "fat" calories. So, I keep peanut butter out of my kitchen—and I make sure to have plenty of low-fat alternatives on hand.

That's the kitchen you want—one with alternatives.

Dealing with Your Kids or an Uncooperative Spouse

As I'm sure you know, it's not always easy to create a low-fat kitchen, especially when you have kids clamoring for those peanut butter sandwiches or when you have a spouse who openly scoffs at your low-fat crusade. Let me offer you a suggestion: Don't rush off and try to convert your whole family to the low-fat life. Such a huge task will lead only to greater stress than you can handle. For now, designate one big shelf in your pantry and one area in your refrigerator as "your" area. That's the place where you will go when you are hungry and when you create your meals. Whenever you are hungry, concentrate on your area, even if you find yourself cooking fried chicken for the rest of your family. This might seem hard to believe, but in time, as long as you stay patient, you'll discover that your family will adapt to the low-fat life.

Learn to Shop

Before we can start the 21-day program, we need to go shopping. And as your personal trainer, I want to take you on a tour of your local grocery store, department by department, and show you exactly what you should buy. In fact, you might want to take this book to your grocery store, open it to this page, and follow my instructions.

When you go to the supermarket, get in the habit of shopping the perimeter of the store. All the natural foods are on the perimeter. That's where you'll find produce, meats and fishes, and low-fat dairy products.

Eat before you food shop. Shopping when you're hungry can lead you to choose the wrong foods almost without thinking about it.

In the inner aisle, you'll find the processed, canned, and frozen foods. I'm not naive. I know this is no longer a society that prepares most of its food from scratch. And I know that you are going to buy food you can pour right out of the can or box. That's fine with me! Sure, fresh food has a higher nutritional value, and it doesn't have as much salt—but listen, canned vegetables are better than no vegetables at all, and they are better than ordering French fries at your nearest fast-food restaurant.

All you really want to do as you begin this program is start finding better choices for the same kinds of food you eat. If you do that alone, you will be launching a major attack on your fat cells.

Watch the Labels

What will really help you is to learn to read nutrition labels, which are required by the Food and Drug Administration to be displayed on most foods. While these "Nutrition Facts" look a little different from the labels you may be used to, they make the fat content of foods and other information very accessible.

But they also can be a little misleading if you aren't careful. For example, when you see a product that says it's "Light" or "Lite," that only means that product contains one-third fewer calories than usual—which could still mean that you are taking in a lot of "fat calories." If a product's label says "Low Fat," that only means you are getting up to three grams of fat per serving, which can also mean a substantial number of "fat calories." I'm not saying to ignore that food—it's better to choose that version than the higher-fat version—but so many people think they are doing all they need to do just by filling up their grocery carts with products that say "low fat."

Here's another commmon mistake: People buy "2 percent milk" believing they are getting only a small percentage of fat in their milk. No. They're only getting 2 percent less fat than what's in whole milk. And guess how much fat is in whole milk? Almost half of the calories that come from a glass of whole milk—49.2 percent—are "fat calories."

And where do "fat calories" go once they get inside

your body? That's right. Your fat cells! If you drink 2 percent milk, you're still getting more than 40 percent fat—and that's way, way too much.

My recommendation is to look for food that has no more than 20 percent of fat per serving. That allows for a surprising amount of room. Obviously, if the label says "fat-free" or "calorie-free," then you're in great shape. (By government definition, calorie-free means no more than 5 calories per serving, and fat-free means no more than 0.5 grams of fat per serving.)

Sometimes, however, the label is not clear about the percentage of "fat calories" you're getting per serving. So here's the way to figure it out when you're looking at a label:

1. Look for the part of the label that discusses the number of calories per serving size. Divide the "Calories from Fat" number by the number that corresponds to total calories in the serving size.

2. You will get a number like 0.25 or 0.30 or 0.15. Take that number, and multiply it by 100. This figure is the percentage of calories that comes from fat.

Here's an example of how to do it. If the label says there are 90 calories in a serving and 30 of those are "calories from fat," then divide 30 by 90 and you get 0.33. Then multiply that figure by 100, converting it to 33 percent. Such a food would not be considered low-fat because of the high percentage of calories that come from fat.

What to Start Buying

In no particular order, I want to give you a long list of items that you can purchase at a grocery store that will help the program work for you. Don't feel you need to memorize this list. Every time you shop, just come back to it and get an idea of what's the best food to buy.

I am a big believer in making grocery shopping fun. I promise you, the grocery store will never become a burden under this program. There are so many great items to choose from that your new low-fat shopping spree will truly be an adventure.

Produce

You can pretty much follow the lists of starchy carbs and fibrous vegetables that I gave you in the previous chapter. Let me throw my favorites at you again. The fresh vegetables to buy are carrots, spinach, peppers, cucumbers, onions, mushrooms, squash, lettuce, asparagus, celery, tomatoes, garlic, cabbage, broccoli, baking potatoes, sweet potatoes, corn, green beans, yams, zucchini, tomatoes, cauliflower, eggplant, and brussels sprouts. Examples of beans to buy would be red beans, kidney beans, black beans, pinto beans, black-eyed peas, sweet peas, and green peas. Grains would be brown rice, basmati rice, wild rice, oats, wheat berries, couscous, corn, barley, buckwheat groats, millet, bulgur, whole corn grits, and many more.

Fruit

It's easy to get confused about fruit. A lot of you look at fruit as this incredible secret weapon for weight loss. But for all of its benefits—it's fibrous and has great nutrients—it doesn't promote weight loss. The calories that come from fruit are easily stored as fat. I'm not saying to avoid fruit. It's like nature's candy—a perfect snack. But just be moderate about your fruit intake, and look for fruits that are lower in sugar than others. The lower-sugar fruits are strawberries, apples, pears, and berries. A little higher in sugar, but still okay, are grapefruit, cantaloupe, mangos, tangerines, oranges, honeydew, papayas, plums, and nectarines. Fruits like bananas, pineapples, peaches, grapes, and watermelon are highest in sugar, but of course, they can still be a part of your eating program. Beware of dried fruits. They are loaded with sugar calories—yes, even the all natural varieties. Fruit is a snack, not a meal substitute.

Meat and Fish

Here are your best meats: boneless, skinless turkey breast; white-meat chicken; white-meat fishes; lean venison and game meats; the very leanest cuts of beef, such as sirloin, eye of round steak, and roast beef; and center-cut pork tenderloin. Canned tuna, white-meat chicken, or white-meat turkey packed in water are also great, but keep reading the labels.

If you can afford it, always buy boneless and skinless chicken breasts; otherwise, make sure you take the time to remove the skin and bones when you cook chicken, because you'll be removing a lot of fat. Another tip: White meat has less fat than dark meat. Dark-meat chicken is over 40 percent fat, while white-meat chicken is only 4 percent fat.

You might be surprised to know that turkey breasts are leaner than chicken. For variety, try the 99 percent fat-free ground turkey. (All other kinds of ground turkey contain parts which are higher in fat.) When it comes to beef, even the leanest is 30 to 35 percent fat. A T-bone steak or a hamburger has up to 60 percent fat. So stick with the leaner cuts.

It's also hard to go wrong with fish—as long as it's white fish. White fish such as cod, flounder, haddock, scrod, halibut, shrimp, mussels, lobster, and crab meat are the least fatty and are loaded with protein. Despite rumors to the contrary, shellfish are no higher in calories than regular fish. However, don't rely too much on darker meat fishes such as salmon, which has 44 percent fat (even though it's considered a better kind of fat than the usual fat you eat). It's astonishing, isn't it, how careful you have to be.

Finally, just in case you're still tempted when you head through the meat section, keep saying to yourself that hot dogs, pork lunch meats, and ground beef are over 50 percent fat. Even though turkey and chicken franks are proclaimed to be lower in fat than a beef frank, they still contain eight to eleven grams of fat each. There are lower-fat Canadian bacon products on the market, which are good for pizza and breakfast. And if you must keep hot dogs in your house, there are now fat-free hot dogs. These items are highly processed, which means high in calories, and they are high in sodium.

Another caution when it comes to deli meats: All deli meats are processed, which means you don't get the same high quality of protein from, say, deli turkey as you do from regular turkey. But some deli meats are better than others. Look for deli meat that is lower in fat and sodium.

Dairy Products

I'm a big lover of cheese—but I learned early on that if I wanted to get lean, I had to get my diet to the point where dairy products such as cheese and milk were treats, not staples. It's virtually impossible to lose significant weight while consuming most cheeses or milk with 1 percent or higher fat content.

Yet with that in mind, the good news is that there are now plenty of great substitutions for high-fat dairy products in the dairy case. Remember how nonfat cheese used to taste like rubber? You couldn't melt it in a microwave. The nonfat cheese today is ten times more delicious. You'll find skim milk, nonfat sour cream, nonfat yogurt, nonfat cottage cheese, nonfat cream cheese, fat-free cheese singles, fat-free Egg Beaters® and egg whites (which are important because all of the fat of an egg is in the yolk—the white has pure protein and no fat).

You've got low-fat butters and margarines, but many of you don't like the taste. Still, you need to break your dependence on butter. It's a killer, even in small doses. I buy something called "I Can't Believe It's Not Butter"® spray. Even though there is a little fat in the product, you consume a lot less fat by spraying as opposed to pouring or spreading.

Freezer Foods

There are some very nutritional frozen foods, from frozen berries to frozen vegetables to frozen turkey and chicken breasts to fat-free waffles and fat-free frozen hash browns (bake them instead of fry them and you won't be able to tell the difference). Lean Cuisine® and Healthy Choice® entrées are not bad, but as I'll explain as we progress through the book, you need to be careful about overusing those kinds of low-calorie dinners.

Processed Foods

In my book, this means anything that comes in a package—from cold cuts, crackers, chips, packaged macaroni, frozen waffles, pancake mixes, pastas, white flour products, cereal, and bread. Some processed foods are good sources of starchy carbs, but by the time they are mixed, mashed, and boxed, they become calorically dense. Your body can't handle them all. Almost all processed foods have loads of added oil, sodium, or sugar.

I don't want you to think that breads, pastas and cereals are bad for you. They're just extremely high in calories. One serving of pasta, which is merely two ounces, contains 210 calories, which is about 50 more calories than a medium-sized baked potato. But very few people sit down to a two-ounce helping of pasta. The plate usually put in front of you consists of six to eight ounces. That's when pasta becomes a poor choice if you want to lose weight. Likewise, bread is one of the first things you need to reduce if you are serious about getting lean. A bagel is so packed with condensed flour that just one of them can contain more than 400 calories! One plain bagel (without any jelly or butter or cream cheese) has as many calories as ten egg whites and a cup of oatmeal.

But let me repeat, I'm not telling you to cut out all processed foods. If you use them in moderation, especially the fat-free varieties, you'll still see weight loss results.

"Health" Foods

Just because a food is classified as a "health" or "natural" food doesn't mean you get lean by eating it. Natural peanut butter, for example, has more fat than regular peanut butter. Six ounces of tofu contain a whopping sixteen grams of fat. Granola is ridiculously high in fat as well. And you have to watch some plant foods. Avocados, coconuts, olives, nuts, and seeds are mostly 80 percent fat. A dried fruit such as raisins has 210 calories per half-cup. So be careful.

Dressings, Sauces, and Oils

Try to keep oil to a bare minimum. That includes salad dressing, vegetable cooking oils, cooking sprays, butter, mayonnaise, sour cream, and margarine. It's oil that makes fried food so fattening, which is why you should stay away from anything fried. A single tablespoon of that oil contains 120 calories of fat—a single tablespoon! If you must use oil, look for oil that claims to be either "monosaturated" or "polyunsaturated," but remember, the less oil the better.

Meanwhile, there are so many different nonfat condiments and spices to add flavor to your food that I could fill an entire refrigerator with nothing but these products. To name a few: Tabasco®, picante sauce, yellow and Dijon mustards, seasoned vinegars, balsamic and wine vinegars, canned tomato paste, horseradish, canned fat-free sauces, fat-free dressings, teriyaki and soy sauces, fat-free taco seasoning mixes, fat-free onion soup mixes, and many more.

If you are not using fat-free dressings because of your memory of how bad they tasted when they were first introduced, try them again. They are now surprisingly tasty.

Desserts

You want to start eliminating food that contains what are known as "simple sugars." These are sugars found in all forms of desserts, and they are called "simple" because they don't need to be broken down by your body. They go straight into your bloodstream and usually right into your fat cells. That's why calories from desserts are called "empty calories." They have no nutritional value.

Nevertheless, you can still find great desserts which are sugar free and fat free. The key for me is to be very careful and eat only one helping of dessert. Just like fat-free snacks, you think you can get away with a second fat-free dessert bar, and boom! You're taking in way too many calories. Small cookies that proclaim to be low fat are deceptively easy to consume. How many times, for example, have you started with one nonfat cookie and ended up eating everything in the box? And you must be alert to sugary products that say they are fat free. Read the labels. I see lots of six-ounce "fat-free" yogurts in the grocery store that also contain twenty-nine grams of sugar. That's the equivalent of seven tablespoons of raw sugar. Can you imagine sitting down and eating seven tablespoons of sugar? I've even seen one eight-ounce fat-free yogurt that is promoted as being deliciously low fat but actually has forty-one grams of sugar!

If you decide to have a dessert, sugar-free and fat-free puddings, Popsicles, and ice creams are the better choices. There are now even fat-free ice cream syrups and toppings. But please, think moderation. What I often do is buy hard candies that are fat free. One or two of them can sometimes help curb a sweet tooth.

Snacks

The number of low-fat salty snacks like chips and crackers on the market these days is fairly overwhelming. But don't overdo it. Just because a product is low fat or fat free doesn't mean it is not loaded with calories. You'll think you can eat lots of the stuff because it's low fat, and you'll find yourself gaining weight because you had no idea how many calories you were actually stuffing into your mouth. What's more, these are hardly the calories that go to your muscle tissue.

However, if you're going to snack, there are some good choices. The plain popcorn that you microwave or use with an air popper is the best. Make sure it's not prepared with cooking oil or says "natural flavored." ("Natural-flavored" popcorn usually has as much fat as butter flavored.) Also, try to get snack boxes that package individual helpings so you're more likely to eat less.

I do not particularly care for the no-fat chips made with fat substitutes like Olestra®—I don't like the greasy aftertaste—so I still go with baked low-fat chips and occasionally dab them in a fat-free bean dip. If you can't stand the new breed of low-fat chips and desperately need a salty snack, go with pretzels. I also buy rice cakes, but I am very careful about them. The flavored rice cakes can have five grams of sugar per serving; five or six rice cakes can suddenly add up to six teaspoons of sugar.

Beverages

If you haven't tried it, then buy some bottled water. As I'll later explain, water is a critical part of the Slimdown for Life. And you don't even have to tell me you don't drink enough water. Few people do. But as weird as this sounds, people do start drinking water if they buy it bottled or flavored. Although tap water is just fine, having bottled water around is more appealing to some people. You can flavor your water with a variety of sugar-free powdered flavors (like Crystal Lite®). I also suggest you stock up on noncaloric drinks when you get bored with water and need a change. Any noncaloric soft drink is fine. But do not be fooled by "sports drinks." They are not necessary for our fitness program, and they are loaded with sugar. Fruit juices are basically water loaded with sugar. If you want fruit, eat the real thing so you can get the fiber.

Soft Drinks, Alcohol, and Coffee

If you do drink a diet soft drink, don't think you're getting your water needs met. Anything with caffeine in it, like colas or coffee, acts like a diuretic. For every cup of caffeinated beverage you have, you need an extra cup of water just to ensure your body is getting enough fluid.

What's more, just because something is liquid doesn't mean it can't go to your fat cells. A twelve-ounce can of nondiet soda, for instance, has forty grams of sugar. What does that mean to you? Divide forty grams by four (which is the number of sugar grams in a teaspoon) and you have *ten* teaspoons of sugar. Could you ever imagine yourself sitting down to eat ten teaspoons of table sugar, most of which would race to your fat cells? Well, you do it all the time. And fruit juices have more sugar, ounce per ounce, than soda does. So cut back. If you reduce just one or two sodas a day along with a big glass of orange juice, and you cut back from three beers on the weekend to two, you're knocking a lot of calories out of your program.

I'm also sure I don't have to warn you about the high sugar content of alcoholic drinks and the incredible number of empty calories in mixed drinks and cream-based liqueurs. I'm not telling you to cut out alcohol, but don't try to justify regular drinking of alcohol by referring to a couple of studies that have come out saying alcohol helps your heart. Alcohol will get you fat in a hurry. Besides the high calories, it acts as a depressant, which means you usually won't want to do a thing the next day, except eat fattening foods you think will make you feel better. Furthermore, you tend to want to eat fat when you drink. Have you ever been to a restaurant, convinced you were going to eat well, and then ate everything in sight after having downed a margarita or glass of wine? At this point, you could care less what you eat after a drink or two. Alcohol can seriously mess up your decision making.

Now, I will tell you, a beer or a glass of wine at night isn't going to ruin your program. If you choose to drink, however, opt for the lower-calorie beverages like wine spritzers and light beer. Ideally, you should try to limit your drinking to special occasions.

I know caffeine is a vice. Too much caffeine causes the excessive release of antistress hormones in your body—and eventually, the body's supply of those hormones becomes depleted. That's when you get headaches and feel fatigue and irritability. But I'm not a tyrant. I drink coffee and caffeinated diet sodas, and I will never tell you to cut those out entirely. Yes, your body's metabolism would run at absolute peak efficiency if you drank only water and kept all caffeine out of your system. But caffeine won't cause you to gain weight, and as long as you are moderate with it, you'll be fine.

Final Purchase

There's one last thing you should buy—a bottle of champagne to celebrate the new body that you will have at the end of the 21-day program! That day is not far away. You now have educated yourself on what it takes to get lean, and you have created the environment around you to allow you to get lean.

Now it's time to go for it, for there is nothing that can hold you back. Right now, all that it takes to attain your goal is for you simply to believe in yourself.

Part Two

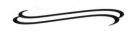

The 21-Day Slimdown for Life Program

Focus on progress, not perfection.

3

Introducing the 21-Day Program

How You'll Use This Book for the Next Three Weeks

This is a program about progress, not perfection.

I don't recommend reading this book like a novel where you can't wait to get to the end. Don't read all twenty-one days in a row. This is a book to be read one day at a time. Read Day One, follow my instructions, listen to my advice, and then shut the book. During your second day on the program, read Day Two, then shut the book again. There's no reason to take in more information than you're actually going to use for that day. Of course, you can go back and review anything from the previous days as often as you wish. After Day Seven, for instance, you might want to go back and read again through the earlier days to pick up little tips and tidbits that you perhaps didn't get the first time you read it.

You can also repeat these twenty-one days over and over and over again, in any way you wish. You can repeat the first week a few times until you think you've got it. Or you can repeat Days Fourteen through Twenty-one. This book is designed to work with you to achieve your leanness goal.

With each week, you will take a significant step forward. Here's how:

Week One: In the first week, you will start off mastering the basic building blocks of the Slimdown for Life. You'll learn the importance of meal frequency, the need to combine the right balance of foods in each meal in order to speed up your body's metabolism, and the need for Sixty-Second Workouts and walking routines. Every day, you will be asked to follow the meal plans and the workouts. You won't be asked to eat and exercise perfectly the first week—far from it. You just want to get started.

Week Two: In the second week, you will start refining your eating and exercise program so it becomes a natural, integral part of your life. This is also the week when, according to those who have gone through the program, you'll really start noticing your body's metabolism changing. Moreover, during this week you'll begin working on another part of your body—your mind. I have often been told that the mental tips you'll be getting are one of the great joys about this program. Besides losing weight, you will learn to work on your mind so that you can stay focused and motivated.

Week Three: In the third week, you will put it all together. For the final seven days, you'll realize the thrill of eating right while simultaneously getting your body into shape. You will start seeing the pounds coming off almost automatically. You won't have to depend anymore on "willpower" to consciously deprive yourself of calories. And you will have the mind-set that will inspire you to get the right food into your body that will slip past your fat cells and rush straight to your muscle tissue.

Just Trust the Program

You might find yourself asking questions during the first several days, feeling confused, wondering why so many things I'm saying go against all the usual stuff you have heard about losing weight. All that I ask you to do is: *Trust the program.*

Considering that almost everyone quits regular diets after two weeks, what is the harm in following my program for the same amount of time? I won't even ask you to stick with me the whole twenty-one days. Just give me two weeks—a mere fourteen days out of your life. Two weeks! This is all that I have asked hundreds of other people who were once skeptics as you might be. I have said, "See how you feel after those two weeks— and if you don't want to go on for the third week, I understand, and I wish you the best."

Then I sit back and wait, because I know what's going to happen. I have hundreds of testimonials from people who say they could tell, after just a few days, that the Slimdown for Life "felt right." Because they were eating the right amounts of proper food, several times a day, they realized they would never again have to pretend to "hate" food or worry about a lack of "willpower."

Ask yourself: Is it worth fourteen days of your life to feel that you were getting healthier *while* you were losing weight? What would it feel like to know that you were eating your way to a lean body rather than trying to "diet" fifty pounds away? And what would it feel like to know that you were eating more food than you ever thought was "allowable"?

All right, it's time to get to work. Let's go to Week One.

CHAPTER

4

Week One

To lose weight, you must prepare your mind as well as your body.

The first thing we're going to do on the Slimdown for Life might seem a little odd. I want you to find a pencil or pen and write down what I call a Personal Mission Statement.

"Mission statements" are used by corporations all the time. They lay out a statement that clearly defines their philosophy and their goals. It can be a wonderful tool for you, too—a way to stay committed to your new life and new body. After you write your own Personal Mission Statement, I recommend that you stick it on your refrigerator door or your bathroom mirror, so it will always be there to remind you to make sure you are headed in the right direction. It is there to remind you that if you try to be the best you can be as a human being, then everything else will follow. Whenever you feel yourself stray, your Personal Mission Statement will be there to get you back on track.

Here's a great example of a Personal Mission Statement that came from someone who had got on the Slimdown:

My mission in life is to attain a state of vibrant physical health that allows me to feel confident and attractive in front of others. I am committed to losing enough weight so that I can live my life with great joy and display the kind of energy that will bring me friends, happiness, and tremendous success.

Now it's your turn. Don't think of this as a test that you have to get right the very first time. Don't worry if it sounds too vague. You can refine this statement over the next weeks and months as often as you want.

My Personal Mission Statement

_____

_____

_____

_____

_____

_____

_____

Is it possible to achieve the goal in your mission statement? I know it is. I have watched it happen time after time after time: people creating a truly unshakable belief in themselves.

Now it's your turn.

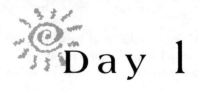

Day 1

Meal Frequency

Welcome, everyone, to your first day on the Slimdown for Life—and let me tell you, you're not going to believe how easy this first day is going to be.

All you have to do is . . . *eat!*

As I've said, the heart of the Slimdown for Life is eating. You eat to lose weight. The first secret to the Slimdown for Life eating program is to eat more often in regular intervals.

Today, you're not going to worry so much about what to eat as when to eat. All you must do today is eat every three to four hours. That's it! You're doing far more good for yourself than you know. Indeed, researchers have discovered that when people take the same amount of food that they eat in their three regular meals—regardless what that food is—and divide it into five meals, they start losing weight. Isn't that amazing? Just by sequencing your meals, spreading them out, you can start dropping weight *without ever changing the food you eat!*

The Power of Frequent Meals

Why are frequent meals so important? Although your goal is to get as much good food as you can past your fat cells and into your lean muscle tissue, you must be wary: Your lean muscle tissue can handle only a certain amount of food at a time. In other words, after you eat that amount, the cells in your muscles shut their doors and don't allow any more food in, no matter how nutritious it is, until it has burned up the food already there. So where does the excess food go? You guessed it. Straight to your fat cells.

Let me give you an example of what I'm talking about. (I'm going to be mentioning calories here, but I'm doing so only to illustrate my point—not to make you think you have to count calories to succeed in this program.) Let's say it's lunchtime, and you have the type of body that needs 500 calories to keep functioning until your next meal. But then you sit down at lunch and ingest enough food to add up to 1,000 calories. That excess 500 calories (no matter where it is coming from—chicken, fruit, or cookies) is most likely to be stored as fat.

Are you getting the picture? If, at some point during the day, you eat a very large meal (which almost all of you do), you're liable to saturate your fat cells. And don't think you're doing yourself a favor if you overeat at one meal and then wait several hours before eating another meal. By then, it's too late. Your body has already taken the extra calories from that first meal and sent them to its fat cells. What's more, all that you're doing by waiting several hours to eat again is to build up your appetite to the point that you'll almost certainly overeat the next time. In fact, your fat cells will play a vicious game with you if you try to lose weight by undereating. The more meals you try to skip in the hope of losing weight, the more your fat cells, sensing an oncoming famine, will send out those notorious enzymes in order to grab most of those calories that you ingest when you finally eat again.

Moreover, when you spend too much time between meals, your body isn't going to want healthful food. Every study done of eating patterns has found that the longer you wait between meals, the greater the amount of high-fat food you will consume at the next meal. Let's say you're trying to get lean, and you have a cup of coffee and toast for breakfast. Then you eat a salad and yogurt for lunch. Then you go from 1:00 P.M. to 7:00 P.M. without eating. When you walk into the house, exhausted and hungry, what do you think you're going to want to eat? Certainly not a healthful meal, like a grilled chicken breast with steamed broccoli and brown rice. You are craving fatty foods and sugar—the very things your muscles will never take in.

This craving is a physical need, not just a psychological one. Your body is shutting down and requires energy in a hurry—and sugar and fat are two of the best ways to get that quick fix. Another reason you crave fat is because you want food that is instantly satisfying, that fills you up fast. It's a fact: Undereating always leads to overeating. Skipping meals will set off an increased craving in your body for the very foods that you're trying to avoid.

How Can You Eat So Often?

Now let me stop and guess what your thoughts might be right at this moment. You think there is no way you can eat so much food four or five times a day. And you believe there is no way you can even find the time to squeeze in so many meals a day.

The fact of the matter is that most of you are already eating five times a day. There's no question about it. What many of you are conveniently ignoring is the caloric impact of your little sixty-second "snacks" that you have in the midmornings and midafternoons. You're also forgetting about that quick graze in front of the refrigerator right before you go to bed at night. You don't realize that those little snacks are usually so high in fat and so loaded with calories that you might as well be eating a full meal.

Let's consider the typical American diet. Doughnuts or a couple of bagels in the morning, then lunch, then some vending machine stuff in the afternoon, a big dinner, and then ice cream late at night. That's five meals. And as you're going to learn tomorrow, if you ate that many times a day, eating all the right foods, you'd be overwhelmed by the amount of food you could eat—and you'd be even more overwhelmed by the fact that you'd start losing weight.

Your Day One Eating Guide

So your task for Day One is very basic. You're not going to find any recommendations on what to eat; that will start tomorrow. I only want you to eat five meals today, each one coming approximately every three to four hours.

Please note: I'm giving you five meals each day because I count the snacks you're eating already as meals. (Considering the kind of quick food you probably eat during a normal snack, a snack is almost always higher in fat and often higher in calories than a regular meal.) Moreover, if you ever happen to note the times you eat during an average day, you will probably realize that when you include your snacks, you might be eating *more* than five times a day.

Another critical point to remember: This week, your

third meal and fifth meal will look more like snacks and low-fat desserts. By next week, however, we will make those into light protein-carb meals just like the others.

I'm offering you times of the day you can eat, but again, I want this program to provide flexibility. You can decide when to have your first meal. Just make sure that you start eating in regular intervals after you finish that first meal. For instance:

Meal One: 8 A.M. Eat your regular breakfast.

Meal Two: 12 P.M. Eat your regular lunch.

Meal Three: 3 P.M. Eat a snack.

Meal Four: 6 P.M. Eat your regular dinner.

Meal Five: 9 P.M. Eat a late-night snack.

Evening Pep Talk

I know that for those of you who have spent much of your adult lives trying out fad diets, I might sound a little bit off the wall. You are still stuck to that wildly outdated theory that our days should consist of three meals—breakfast, lunch, and dinner. But what I'm giving you is the result of reports from the top researchers in the field who have studied permanent weight loss and determined exactly what it takes to get fat off your body forever.

Some of you are probably wondering what I'm holding back. I'm not holding back a thing. This is what true progress is all about. It's about moderation and balance. It's about creating small daily habits that will give you the ability to eat well for the rest of your life. You will never turn back once you see your body change.

Slimdown Tip: Slow Down Your Eating

You can make surprising changes in your eating behavior just by slowing down the speed at which you eat. A lot of people who eat too much of the wrong foods don't even know what they're eating because of how quickly they race through their meals. Today, time yourself and see if you're taking a bite of food every five or ten seconds. Ideally, you want to do it somewhere between fifteen and thirty seconds—and if you can hold out longer, so much the better.

Keep this in mind, too: Your brain needs about twenty minutes to recognize that you have eaten enough to satisfy your body's needs. So if you eat more slowly during this twenty-minute period, you'll consume less food but feel equally satisfied at the end of those twenty minutes as compared to faster eaters who will consume much more food in those first twenty minutes but not have any idea how full they are until much later, when they can barely move off the couch.

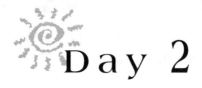

Day 2

The Sixty-Second Workout

Today is another easy day. You will be continuing to work on your meal frequency, and you are going to add a couple of exercises to make your muscle tissue burn calories far more efficiently. All you have to do is two workouts today that last no more than sixty seconds each.

For those of you who haven't worked out in a long time, don't be afraid of the word "muscle." Muscle is the best calorie-burning tissue the body has, and when the muscles are called into action, their calorie-burning ability can increase as much as twentyfold. And listen to me: You can get those results without having to use barbells. You don't have to do ten reps while lying in a prone position under a bulky bench-press machine. You do not—I repeat, do not—need to devote several afternoons a week putting on workout clothes and going to a gym, spending an hour working up a sweat, then showering, dressing again, and going home.

The Easy Truth About Muscle Training

I admit, I was once a bodybuilder wannabe. I devoted my life to the gym. My workouts today are a lot easier and lot shorter—and I don't feel I am missing a thing. I want to let you in on a little secret. If you closely watch a big-time weightlifter do a series of repetitions with weight, you'll notice that the time he is actually lifting is about sixty seconds or less before he takes a long rest.

Essentially, that's what you'll be doing—except you won't be producing the stereotypical "pumping iron" muscle. This will be lean, silky, beautiful muscle. You'll be taking your long-dormant skeletal muscle tissue, which right now probably feels like fat, and you'll be rebuilding its elasticity and tone.

I can't tell you how many of my old-school colleagues give me a hard time about the idea of my Sixty-Second Workouts. They say, "Oh, come on, who can get in shape in sixty seconds?"

And I always reply, "I've met a lot of people who have turned their lives around with just one Sixty-Second Workout. As time passes, they add more Sixty-Second Workouts each day. I know people who were unable to get through thirty seconds of a Sixty-Second Workout, and a few weeks later were doing a dozen of them a day."

Despite all the huffing and puffing you see people doing at health clubs, the truth is that the most elementary resistance exercise—from leaning one arm against the wall to placing your two hands together and pushing—stimulates the kind of muscle activity that can burn calories. It's not the weight you use that counts, it's how you use the weight. That's one of the beauties of the Slimdown for Life. Rather than being inundated with a lot of restrictive instructions on how to work your biceps, triceps, and abs, you only need to use your body weight on some simple exercises. In later weeks, you occasionally might use cans from your pantry as dumbbells, and—who knows?—somewhere down the road you might join a gym. But that's up to you. All you have to do in this program are quick, easy exercises that you will always be able to fit into your schedule.

In the exercise section toward the end of the book, you'll see photos and descriptions of the Sixty-Second Workouts. Some work your upper body, some your lower body, and there are others that stretch your muscles, giving you the critical elasticity to keep your muscle tissue vibrant.

Your Day Two Workout

For today, your goal is to complete two Sixty-Second Workouts. Let's do an upper-body and lower-body workout. (As we continue through the program, I will not require you to do any specific workouts. In this program, any muscle-building exercise, regardless of where it is on the body, is going to get results.)

The first workout for you to do is what I call the "Modified Push-up." Instead of being on the ground doing the far more difficult Marine-style push-up, this is a push-up you can perform from your desk at work or the kitchen counter or dining room table. Stand about three feet away from the desk or table. Then lean forward at an angle and place your hands, which should be shoulder-width apart, against the object. Do push-ups for about sixty seconds—or as long as you can last. The more slowly you perform the push-ups, the better your workout will be.

Now, let's do a lower-body workout: "Standing Heel Raises." Stand with your feet together, go up on your toes, and then come down, letting your heels just barely touch the ground. Then repeat over and over for sixty seconds—or as long as you can last.

If you were laughing before at the idea of Sixty-Second Workouts, I bet you aren't laughing now. I doubt very many of you are able to go the entire sixty seconds. That's normal. Now do you realize what kind of workout you can do in that short space of time?

Your Day Two Eating Guide

Are you continuing to spread out your meals evenly? If you are the type who has tried all your life to eat twice a day at most, you're probably wondering if you can make yourself eat every three hours. All I want you to do is try. Add meals, whatever they are. You have to get yourself into the routine of meal frequency. If you are the type who nibbles and eats all the time, then try to limit yourself to five specific mealtimes, every three hours. Don't get impatient and think there is so much more to do. Just by spreading out your meals, you are reconditioning your body to lose weight.

Let me again show you how to spread out your meals:

Meal One: Your regular breakfast.

Meal Two: Your regular lunch.

Meal Three: An afternoon snack.

Meal Four: Your regular dinner.

Meal Five: A late-night snack.

Evening Pep Talk

There's no other way around it: To make your muscle cells work more efficiently, you've got to work them out.

Allowing a muscle to go unused not only compromises your health, but it also keeps you from full physical potential. Not as much blood travels through an unused muscle, which means that muscle won't get enough oxygen and calcium, which means your tendons and ligaments become fragile. Eighty percent of all lower back pain may be attributed to muscular deficiency. And studies also show that those who do not do any kind of muscle toning are more likely to develop osteoporosis—a condition in which your bones weaken and you start to hunch over as you get older.

And if you're worried that you're going to look like a bodybuilder, forget it. Research professors on women's health have verified that a basic resistance exercise program—i.e., something like the Sixty-Second Workouts—will lead to phenomenal gains in a woman's strength with very little change in the overall size of her muscle. So instead of worrying about your appearance as a result of the Sixty-Second Workouts, you should be celebrating the fact that what you'll see is a decrease in the size of your hips and thighs because of the significant amount of fat that you'll lose. You don't get bigger. You only look better. And who can complain about that?

I have no doubt that you are quickly going to realize that your time to exercise is so precious in your life. But like everything else, don't overdo your workouts. Relax. More weight is not great. You don't gain through pain. To me, pain only means one thing—you're hurting. And I think by now you know all too well that if you feel pain or burn out too quickly, then you're going to call it quits.

Slimdown Tip: Vitamins

My feelings about vitamins have flip-flopped in the past few years. I once believed that you should take everything that was made, from liver tablets to protein powders to super-megavitamin packets. Then I went through a phase where I felt no vitamins were necessary. Today, I believe that vitamins have a place— as long as they are used in moderation and not as substitutes for healthful eating. Here's what I would do: Take a good multiple vitamin or packet of vitamins as recommended. It's a great addition to your program, because even with the best eating, you could still use some added vitamins. For those of you who are vegetarians, a protein supplement such as a protein powder can help.

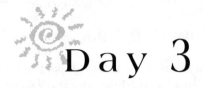

Day 3

The Balanced Meal

Today, we learn about another cornerstone of the Slimdown for Life: what you will be eating. By the end of the day, you are going to eat one perfectly balanced meal. In the Slimdown for Life, it is imperative you have both a lean protein and a starchy carb at each meal, with a fibrous vegetable thrown in as often as you wish. The lean protein and starchy carb are the two vital elements in your eating program, and you want to do your best to get both on your plate at every meal.

I have no doubt that some of you are already thinking, "Lean proteins, starchy carbs, and fibrous vegetables? You call that appetizing?"

If you recall those lists of foods I have given you, and if you look at the variety of simple recipes in the back of the book and if you study the meals I will be providing for you each day from now on, you'll realize that very little is being removed from your usual choices of foods. You'll only end up preparing or ordering some of those foods differently.

The Need for Balance

Here is the beauty of eating this kind of balanced meal. You will be eating twice the amount of actual food that you usually eat in a typical high-fat meal—and you'll still be taking in *fewer* calories! Let me repeat and repeat and repeat: By eating more of the higher-quality foods, you lose weight faster!

Every time you eat, it is important for you to remind yourself that all calories are not created equal. The calories you get when you eat a French fry are far different from the calories in a baked potato. The science is very clear on this matter. If you eat a bite of food that contains just one gram of fat, then you will have ingested 9 calories (those are called "fat calories"). But food from a gram of starchy carbs provides just 4 calories, and food from a gram of lean protein also has just 4 calories.

Do you realize the implication of these numbers? Here is what you could substitute for two teaspoons of butter: a half-cup of oatmeal, or four egg whites, or two cups of broccoli, or four cups of lettuce, or one and a half cups of air-popped popcorn. That's a lot of food. At the University of Alabama, doctors asked one group of volunteers to eat low-fat foods until they felt full. The doctors then asked another group to eat high-fat foods until they felt full. On the high-fat diet, the volunteers usually started feeling full after having had about 3,000 calories a day. On the low-fat diet, the volunteers started feeling full after eating just 1,570 calories a day.

I was once on a national talk show, and without my knowing it, the producers had prepared five meals that fit the Slimdown for Life. They rolled all the meals out on a table in front of me.

The hosts kept staring at the food, and then they looked at me dubiously. "You mean to tell us you can eat all this food in one day and actually lose weight?" one of the hosts asked.

"Easily," I said.

The hosts just stared at me.

"I can do it because all the food you're looking at is composed of starchy carbs and lean protein," I said. "And that kind of food doesn't get stored as fat. Do you realize that one Big Mac, a large order of fries, and a chocolate shake have more calories than four grilled chicken breasts, two baked potatoes, two cups of rice, and six cups of fibrous vegetables?"

The hosts' mouths began to drop open.

"And do you know that your twelve-ounce soda and candy bar are equivalent in calories to the ten egg whites, cup of oatmeal, and toast that I eat in the morning?"

The mouths fell open a little farther.

"And here's the kicker. That kind of food you're eating is more inclined to go to your fat cells and make you look fat. My food acts like fuel."

The hosts weren't sure what to say. I think I had made my point.

The lean protein–starchy carb combination is the ideal way to regulate your blood sugar level, to fuel your muscles, and give you the immediate energy to function properly. It keeps you from experiencing sugar cravings that can lead to wild chocolate binges, and it can prevent those insulin-caused peaks and valleys that can make you pig out.

Most important, if you eat the proper balance of starchy carbs and lean proteins at every meal, you are essentially shooting the equivalent of jet fuel into your body, forcing your metabolism to operate at a much more rapid rate! The faster your metabolism, the faster your calories are burned off.

Let's say that you were very conscientious about spacing every meal evenly apart during the day. But in one meal, all you ate were starchy carbs (for instance, a large baked potato), and in another meal it was all protein (chicken the size of your palm), and in another meal it was all fibrous vegetables (a large salad). The problem with this kind of eating is that your muscle tissue will only take in so many carbs and so much lean protein at a time. So if you eat more than the proper amount of starchy carbs or proteins at one meal, your muscle tissue won't be able to absorb it, and off to the fat cells the excess carbs or protein go.

On the other hand, if you don't eat a protein and starchy carb at each meal, your blood sugar might lower too quickly, leading you to binge on high-fat foods. With a balanced eating program, the desire for fat significantly diminishes.

Your Day Three Eating Guide

As I said earlier, we're going to take it slowly as we move into our eating plan. Today, all I want you to do is try to make Meal Four perfectly balanced. As for the other meals, I want you to find ways to cut back your normal intake of fat or at least to substitute slightly better foods for the ones you normally eat.

Below is a list of sample meals. But please take note: *You do not have to eat those foods if you don't like them.* If you hate turkey sandwiches, for example, then come up with a different protein to eat. Forcing yourself to eat foods that you hate is a sure-fire guarantee that you will quit this program before the week is over.

Meal One: Cereal with skim milk, two slices of toast with jam.

Meal Two: A turkey sandwich with mustard (never mayonnaise) and baked chips.

Meal Three: For your afternoon snack, try crunchy vegetables (such as a bag of baby carrots from the grocery store) instead of a candy bar.

Meal Four: Here is your perfectly balanced meal. One chicken fillet grilled with no oil or butter, a baked potato with fat-free cheese, fat-free sour cream, chives, and a salad with fat-free dressing.

Meal Five: For your evening snack, try a bowl of oatmeal (using little or no sugar) instead of something like ice cream.

Your Day Three Workout

Again, it's very simple. You must complete only two Sixty-Second Workouts. For your upper body workout, do a Bicep Curl. Stand with your knees and hips slightly bent to create a slight forward tilt with the upper body. Keep your back straight and shoulders back, and your arms should be straight down and to the side of the body with your elbows slightly bent. Now, raise your lower arms as far as possible without moving your shoulders or upper arms. When you reach the top of the movement, squeeze the biceps, then slowly lower them back down and repeat for sixty seconds. If you wish, you can hold a soup or vegetable can in each hand while performing the exercise for extra resistance.

For your lower-body workout, do the Reverse Lunge. This is a great overall leg exercise. Stand with your feet shoulder-width apart, as if you are standing on railroad tracks, your knees and hips slightly bent. Hold your arms to your sides. Take one foot and step backward as if you're taking one giant step backward in the old Simon Says game. Plant your toe firmly against the ground with the knee only slightly bent. Hold for a couple of seconds, maintaining your balance, and then return to your starting position, keeping your back straight. Then begin again, this time stepping back with the other leg.

Evening Pep Talk

By now, you've done your first Slimdown for Life meal, and I promise you, your fat cells are in trouble. In the coming days, as you add more Slimdown meals to your program and start your exercise program, your body will start going through incredible changes! As long as you follow this program, it will be impossible for you *not* to lose weight!

Slimdown Tip: Determining How Much Food You Need

Here is the standard rule that I follow for men and women: Your protein (such as a piece of lean meat) should be able to fit into your hand, your starchy carb sould be about the size of your fist, and your fibrous vegetable should be able to fit into a small cereal bowl. That's it. If you're a larger person, you might add a little more food—but anyone staying within the above parameters is going to be on track.

You never really have to carry around one of those 500-page books that tell you the calorie content of everything. If you're eating the right kinds of foods at each meal, and if they are approximately the sizes I mentioned, the number of calories and fat grams will take care of themselves. You just have to make sure you're getting the right balance and right proportions of food!

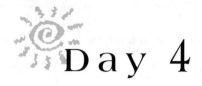

Day 4

Cardio Workout

You've been waiting for this day, haven't you? This is the day, you're thinking, when I exhort you to take up some calorie-blasting, super-fat-burning workout. You think you're going to have to memorize those old phrases: "Go for the burn!" "Let's get physical!"

If there is anything that should make you leap out of bed in the days to come, it's the knowledge that the best cardio program to help you lose weight is one that requires you to go slower!

That's right. Do you remember how I earlier told you about the enzymes in your body that help your fat cells collect calories? Here's the beautiful thing: Your body has other enzymes that can be sent out to take those calories *out* of your fat cells. And a great way to stimulate those enzymes is through *moderate* exercise— and I mean moderate!

Just as fire needs oxygen to burn, so does fat burn in the presence of oxygen. If you work out too hard, you become what is called "anaerobic," which means your body is in "oxygen debt." Because oxygen isn't getting into your fat cells, your body uses its sugar supplies for energy. There's nothing wrong with that—but it's not the most efficient way to lose weight.

It's moderate exercise that gets oxygen into the fat cells, which then sets off a kind of reaction that starts releasing fat calories. You don't need to run a marathon, or sprint as fast as you can as if you're fleeing for your life. You don't need to sweat through your clothes. Indeed, you don't burn extra amounts of fat just because your lungs are gasping for oxygen.

Nor must you work out for an extraordinary length of time when you do cardio exercise. The newest information we have shows that fat-burning exercising can be accomplished in bits and pieces—a few minutes here, a few minutes there. Researchers at the University of Pittsburgh asked two groups of overweight women to walk for a total of forty minutes a day. The first group of women had to walk for forty straight minutes. The second group could divide their forty-minute walks into three daily sessions. The women who divided their forty minutes not only made the same cardiovascular advances as the women who walked all at once, but they also lost an average of five more pounds over the twenty-week period of the study.

Did the Pittsburgh researchers uncover some great mystery about the human body? Actually, they figured something out about human behavior. "The women taking the briefer sojourns were less likely to skip their walks," the study found. "The flexibility associated with exercising in short bouts . . . allowed for more consistent exercise participation."

The Power of Walking

If you take small but consistent steps—a theme that you will hear echoed throughout this book—then you will make great strides in reshaping your body. That's it, ladies and gentlemen. When people ask how much I run, or how many aerobics classes I take, or how long

I ride my bike, I look them square in the eye and say, "I walk. I put on some tennis shoes and I walk."

Walking burns calories just as effectively as running or cross-country skiing or playing a vigorous game of tennis. It only takes a little longer. According to one study, 150-pound women who walked three times a week for an hour automatically lost fifteen pounds—and that's without any change in their food intake. In another study, researchers at the University of Georgia had overweight students and staff do treadmill work, four times a week, expending 300 calories per session. One half did the treadmill work at high intensity, while the other half went much more slowly but for a longer period, to reach the 300-calorie level. Astonishingly, both groups group lost an identical amount of fat—five pounds!

Besides continuing your work on your eating program, all you have to do today is walk around the block. Walk more than once if you wish, but all I'm asking for now is one time around.

You don't want to make your walk a leisurely, casual stroll, but you don't want to walk so fast that you end up huffing and puffing. Throughout your cardio program, if you ever find yourself gasping for breath—indeed, if you can't carry on a normal conversation while walking—then you're going too hard and not burning fat as efficiently as possible.

Is there a voice in you saying, "Oh, come on, Larry! How can you burn enough calories to lose fat by walking around the block?" No doubt you've seen those charts in other books that tell you that doing a triathlon or going cross-country skiing burns a zillion more calories than walking. And of course, you've noticed those great, muscular bodies of professional athletes and have said to yourself, "I've got to work out like that athlete if I want to look like him or her."

Sorry, but you're misleading yourself. The goal here is not to become a professional athlete—nor is the goal to exercise the way you did when you were sixteen years old. *Your goal is to get the physiology of your body to change so that it turns into a far better fat-burning machine.*

You can do any type of cardio you wish. If you want to jog, rollerblade, swim, or take aerobics dance classes, great! But in my program, I'm going to focus on walking because that's what I see the majority of people doing. Even in health clubs filled with extravagantly complicated machines, it's always the treadmills that are in the highest demand. And walking does everything for you that you need to acomplish to get the fat off. As distinguished an institution as the Cooper Institute of Aerobics Research, the Dallas organization that invented the word "aerobics," no longer says that it's intense, vigorous exercise that leads to healthier bodies. The institute's exercise physiologist, Dr. John Duncan, says, "We now know that metabolic changes occur at very moderate exercise intensities."

Did you hear that phrase? Metabolic changes? That's right, you can speed up your valuable metabolism by doing something other than running, other than grunting and groaning, other than leaping around like Michael Jordan. And as I've said over and over, and will continue to say over and over in this book, the speedier your metabolism, the more calories you burn.

Your Day Four Eating Guide

To make egg whites, all you have to do is crack an egg gently in half, and hold one half in one hand and the other half in your other hand. Pour the yellow egg yolk from shell to shell while letting all the egg white drip into a bowl below you. (You want to get rid of the yellow yolk because that's where all the fat is in an egg.) If you're not sure you like egg whites, add two whole eggs to two egg whites to get used to the taste.

Meal One: Try scrambled egg whites (your lean protein) with toast or a bagel. Avoid using butter or oil. Nonstick frying pans are the best for stovetop cooking, but if you don't have one, use a low-fat kitchen spray to lightly coat the pan. (If you prefer an omelette, then make your omelette using only egg whites.)

Meal Two: Try a lean ground beef hamburger or turkey burger (see the recipe chapter) with mustard and ketchup or fat-free mayo.

Meal Three: For your mid-afternoon snack, instead of a bag of potato chips, try three cups of air-popped popcorn. (You can pop it the night before and bring it with you to work.)

Meal Four: Go for a lean red meat like an eight-ounce filet mignon (sixteen ounces is way too much), along with an order of baked or roasted potatoes for your starchy carb. Pick a fibrous veggie of your choice, like spinach.

Meal Five: Go for low-calorie fruit, such as strawberries, apples, pears, or berries. For flavor, add some non-fat whipped cream.

Your Day Four Workout

1. Do two more Sixty-Second Workouts. This time, pick your own.
2. Walk around the block. Suggested time: fifteen to twenty minutes. Don't act like you're wandering in your garden, but don't try to race around the block either. The most effective walking pace, according to researchers, is going over one mile in fifteen minutes. That's about 120 steps a minute. If that speed is too fast for you right now, no problem. Just walk. You'll get there. Remember, you expend the same number of calories walking a mile as you do running a mile. It only takes you longer.

Evening Pep Talk

I hope you realize just how far you progressed today. For those of you who have done no cardio exercise in a very long time, your simple walk probably had the same physical effect on you as a five-mile run does for a conditioned athlete. In that one walk around the block, you got your body's long-dormant furnace going—and it began gobbling up calories far faster than someone who's more conditioned and who has been working out for a long time.

Stay with it. Although I'm not going to ask you to

walk again for a couple of days, you can walk all you want. If you feel yourself get tired and wanting to slow down, then by all means slow down. But at least keep moving. With each step you're taking, you're trans- forming your body into the finely tuned engine it can be. Stop thinking that your body is worn-out and rusted and overweight. Every time you walk, you are stoking your inner furnace. Furthermore, besides sending oxy- gen to the fat cells, exercise sends more oxygen to the brain and makes you feel far more alert throughout the rest of your day in everything you do.

In other words, if you start moving your body, you start changing your life.

Slimdown Tip: Morning Exercise

I have found out that if I wait until later in the day to work out, I usually have so many things that come up on my schedule that I run out of time, or I'm just too exhausted from my workday to do any- thing else except collapse when I get home. So I work out early in the morning, when I am at my freshest.

If you would just set your alarm fifteen or twenty minutes earlier each day, you'd have time to get in all the Sixty-Second Workouts you wanted. If you set it thirty minutes early, you could get in a walk. I know you probably don't like getting up earlier than you have to, but once you do get up, you'll always be glad that you did.

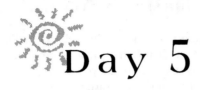

Day 5

Pre-preparing Your Meals

Would you like to know the main reason why people don't get the results they hope for when they try to lead a low-fat life? It's because they don't have the right food available—or are not sure how to get the right food—when it comes time for a meal. They either haven't bought the right food at the supermarket or they haven't pre-prepared their meals in advance.

Well, we're about to change all that. Before you get too involved in the Slimdown for Life, you need to learn to have the right food close by. Considering how often you're going to be eating from now on, you can't hope to succeed if you don't have the food at your fingertips. There's absolutely no way around it. You cannot be leaping up from your desk at the office a couple of times a day to search for the right food. Nor can you afford to put off meals, which will lead to cravings that keep you thinking about food all the time. You never want to find yourself in a position where you are hungry and all you're stuck with is vending machine food or fast food or snacks in the pantry. You don't want to be getting home from work late at night and be so hungry that you start wolfing down whatever you can get your hands on.

When it's time for your meals, you've got to be ready. It doesn't count to have a frozen chicken breast in the freezer or an uncooked potato that will take time to fix.

You will be too hungry to wait. You'll end up snacking on things while you wait for that meal to be cooked, and by the time you're ready to eat, you'll have already downed hundreds of calories that are already on their way to your fat cells.

Have a Couple of Meals Ready

So what am I asking you to do? Spend hours in the kitchen? No, just the opposite. If this begins to feel like a marathon cooking program for you, you'll shut this book in a heartbeat. I want you to learn to have meals ready quickly. Preparing meals before you need them saves you tremendous time and money, and any person with minimal cooking experience can be prepared.

In this book, I'm going to suggest that you always have a couple of meals ready at any given time. That's all you need to do. There are some people I know on this program who pre-prepare a week's worth of the right kind of food. They pop a dozen chicken breasts and/or fish fillets on the grill, put ten baked potatoes in the oven, boil beans and steam vegetables on the stove, make a salad—and then store the food they're going to eat those first three days in the refrigerator, putting the rest in the freezer. After three days, they start taking the food out of the freezer, letting it thaw overnight, and then reheat or microwave it the next day. Bang! They have a meal!

Let me tell you how I pre-prepare meals. The night before, I make a protein–carb meal replacement drink (see today's Slimdown Tip), and then I put that in the refrigerator for my first meal in the morning. Often that same night, I may pre-prepare the next morning's second meal by cracking open eggs and putting the egg whites in a bowl with chopped vegetables. All I have to do is throw the concoction on the stove to make an egg white omelette. I also pull food out of the freezer (something like a grilled piece of lemon-pepper chicken with some rice and steamed broccoli), thaw it, and then carry that meal out of the house with me in a little plastic container.

> Be sure the container you choose to bring to work is microwave proof—just in case you'd like to heat it up. The last thing you want is a meltdown.

Trust me, once you get into the habit of bringing your own food with you each day, it's no different from making sure you have your car keys. There are truck drivers on this program who are on the road so often that they carry coolers full of North-quality food. That way, they can get their meals in all day long.

"But Larry," you're saying, "this is not exactly what anyone would call gourmet eating."

Well, think about your meals and your snacks on a typical day. How many of them last longer than ten minutes? How many of them do you remember ten minutes later? How many of them are magnificent gourmet feasts?

You'll have plenty of opportunities to eat glorious low-fat meals: just look at the recipe chapter. But also remember that the Slimdown for Life, at its core, is a regular eating program. And I'd rather you have pre-prepared some basic foods that you can use for some of your daily meals instead of grabbing some doughnuts in the morning or potato chips in the afternoon and pretend that you're just having a harmless snack. After days and days of those snacks, the weight creeps up on you. To reshape your body, you have to keep injecting it regularly with better fuel, not junk.

Your Day Five Eating Guide

For Day Five, I want you to pre-prepare a meal that you will eat later in the day. Let's make it easy. Grill some extra chicken today, then use some of it for Meal Two (which you'll see below) and some for Meal Three.

Meal One: Try a breakfast shake. Put ice and a banana in a blender with one packet of a meal replacement product (see Slimdown Tip below). Add a little skim milk. Blend until the concoction is creamy, and drink.

Meal Two: Grilled chicken sandwich with lettuce and tomato. Or you could try one of the salads in the recipe section, such as the Fiesta Bean and Corn Salad, sprinkling in some chicken for your protein.

Meal Three: Drop by the grocery store, buy a couple of small bags of crunchy vegetables, and you have your afternoon snack.

Meal Four: For dinner, try a pasta without oil or butter, sprinkle it with slices of chicken that you prepared earlier today, and add a fibrous veggie of your choice.

Meal Five: Try a nonfat ice cream bar.

Your Day Five Workout

Today, we take a big step forward and boost the number of Sixty-Second Workouts. This time, try to do four or possibly five workouts. Pick any five you wish, and make sure to include one or two Sixty-Second Workouts that are in the stretching section.

Also, it's time for your second of three walks for the week. You'll walk fifteen to twenty minutes. Do you know that sucking in your stomach as you walk is a type of sit-up that, over the long run, can tighten your stomach muscles. When walking, lightly swing your arms, keeping your elbows bent at a 90-degree angle. That swinging motion alone will help you walk a little faster and will certainly burn more calories.

Evening Pep Talk

Don't lose patience. We're still adding all the building blocks to the Slimdown. Every little thing you're learning to do now will pay off in a big way later. Here's something to think about. Did you know that each time you drop 10 percent in your body weight, your incidence of heart disease decreases by 20 percent?

That's right. More than 900,000 Americans die of heart disease every year. The reason so many die from heart disease is because of their high levels of cholesterol—which is mainly caused by *excess fat!* With every extra pound of fat you take in, you're adding a lot of extra blood vessels in your body—miles of them. These blood vessels drain away the very blood you need to work through your other body organs. Foods with a high amount of fat can also clog your arteries, which makes it more difficult for blood to circulate.

Every little thing you can do to knock fat out of your body is a great, great victory. You must never forget this. The grim reality is that, over time, fat can kill you. Nearly 90 percent of the 11 million Americans suffering from diabetes have what doctors call Type II diabetes, which is the form most closely associated with excess weight. Did you know if you are an overweight woman, you have a much greater chance of contracting cancer of the uterus or womb, cancer of the ovary, and cancer of the breast? Did you know if you're an overweight man, a high-fat diet puts you at greater risk for prostate and colon cancer?

So give yourself a pat on the back. You're doing far more good for yourself than you even know.

Slimdown Tip: Meal Replacement Products

One way to ensure you get in all your meals each day is by relying on powdered "meal replacement products" that you blend in a glass with iced water and a piece of fruit and drink. In the past, you had to hold your nose to get these drinks down your throat. But now they taste great and provide a good balance of protein and carbohydrates. You can get them now at almost any grocery store.

Clearly, they shouldn't be a major part of your eating program. You always should look for something to "eat." Studies show that if you don't actually get something to chew between your teeth, you'll never feel full no matter how many meal replacement drinks you have a day. Still, I have no objection to them compared to some of the other high-fat foods you can eat. Moreover, the protein in these powders serves as a nice alternative if you get tired of so many protein dishes during the day.

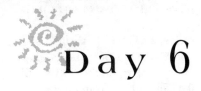

Day 6

Special Ordering

Doing the Slimdown for Life would be a lot easier if you spent all your time inside your house. But in this day and age, most Americans eat away from home an average of four times a week. They spend 40 percent of their monthly food budgets at restaurants. Obviously, you've got to learn to deal with restaurant food and make that food fit into your Slimdown program, or you're not going to succeed.

Restaurants have a way of loading up food with fat. Even some restaurants that offer menus with items that read "healthy heart" or "lite" on them can be misleading. When waiters tell you the cooks use only "a little oil" on the food, you need to be skeptical. It's likely the cooks are in the kitchen drowning the food in oil. They could have marinated their meats in oil and cooked all their vegetables with butter.

Yet regardless what type of restaurant you are in, you can make yourself a low-fat meal. Wherever you are, it's possible to create what I call the North Plate—an order of protein (usually grilled chicken or fish), a starchy carb (perhaps brown rice or a potato dish), and a fibrous vegetable. And you can get a variety of condiments and sauces at the restaurant to enhance flavor. The truth is that you can put together a North Plate at any greasy spoon in town.

First, look the menu over very carefully to see what

foods the restaurant has available. Let's take a burger restaurant. They should have lots of lettuce and tomato to dress up the hamburger. All right, there's your fibrous vegetable. They make french fries from potatoes, so ask very politely if they might have an extra baked potato lying around. Okay, you've got your starchy carb. And almost always, there's a chicken sandwich on the menu. Order that plain (with no mayonnaise and, if you can handle it, with no bread), and there's your protein.

If you are in a place that serves only fried chicken, then pull off the skin. You won't be getting out all the greasy fat that comes with fried foods, but at least you're somewhat ahead of the game. And if they have nothing but hamburgers, then order a hamburger and not a cheeseburger, which again saves you at least something.

Do you see how little substitutions can help you? If you went to a Mexican restaurant and simply ordered grilled chicken fajitas without oil or butter, pico de gallo instead of sour cream, tomato and lettuce instead of cheese, corn tortilla instead of flour tortilla, and extra green and red sauce instead of guacamole, the savings would be enormous. You could keep well over a thousand calories out of your body, at least half of those calories being "fat calories."

And don't ever, ever, ever make the mistake so many people do—which is that cutting back a little item here or there from a higher fat meal isn't going to have any effect on your body. Over time, it will save you a lot of pounds.

How to Place a Special Order

Later in the book, I devote an entire chapter to specific low-fat dishes you can order at specific restaurants—from Chinese to Italian to Mexican to fast food. If you're going to a cafeteria or steak house or even an Indian restaurant, this section will show you what to order. It also will give you an array of techniques when ordering to make sure the kitchen gets the fat out of your food.

But as you get started on this program, I want you initially to focus on a few easy guidelines. All you need is a little knowledge and a little confidence, and restaurants will give you the kind of low-fat meal you want. You're not going to catch every high-fat slip the restaurant makes, of course. But through some simple requests, you can eliminate the equivalent of one shot glass full of cooking oil, another shot glass full of melted butter, another shot glass full of salad dressing, and one full of sugar. That's a lot of fat calories you're knocking out of your diet, especialy if you eat out a lot.

Today, I want you to go out and have a meal at a restaurant, and when you do, follow these easy suggestions:

1. Ask that your entrée (fish, chicken, or beef) be grilled with no oil. That's all you have to say: "Would you cook it with no oil." If the waiter asks you what you want your meat to be cooked in, say lemon or lime juice as an alternative to oil or butter. You would not believe how many hundreds of fat calories you keep out of your body just by doing that.

2. If you think meat cooked in such a way won't be tasty enough, then order a sauce on the side for flavor. But do not—I repeat, do not—spear your food first and then dip it in the dressing. In that case, your food will be slathered with calories. Instead, dip your fork in the sauce and then spear your food. That gives you enough of the flavor you need without getting too many calories.

Do the same thing if you are putting salad dressing on your salad.

3. Ask for vegetables that are steamed, boiled, or sautéed in water. Again, say to the waiter, "Could you make sure the vegetables are not cooked in oil or butter?"

4. Ask the waiter to remove any premeal temptations from your table, such as butter, bread, crackers, or tortilla chips. A premeal roll with butter is the equivalent of a couple of orders of vegetables.

5. Finally, be specific about these requests. You will never feel worse than when you order what you think is a low-fat dish and learn later that it is swamped with fat. For example, you sit down for breakfast in a restaurant and proudly ask for an egg white omelette without cheese. But because you forgot to ask that no oil or butter be used, that omelette could come out swimming in fat. If you'd special ordered it, you would have brought the fat content of that omelette down to almost zero.

6. If they mess up, don't fret. You tried.

Your Day Six Eating Guide

Since we're focusing today on special ordering at restaurants, all five meals are designed to help you at restaurants. I'm not saying to go out and eat every meal at a restaurant today, but depending on what time you are out at a restaurant, here are examples of meals to order. Obviously, when you're at home today, choose meals from the selection I have already given you from the previous five days.

Meal One: Go to a restaurant and order an egg white omelette, cooked without oil, butter, or cheese; include a variety of vegetables in the omelette; then add either dry toast or dry English muffin and a bowl of oatmeal topped with berries or raisins.

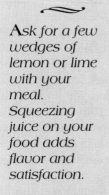

Ask for a few wedges of lemon or lime with your meal. Squeezing juice on your food adds flavor and satisfaction.

Meal Two: Load up on vegetables at a salad bar, but avoid croutons, shredded cheddar cheese, bacon bits, and any of the creamier salads like potato salad or macaroni salad, which can contain an astonishing nine grams of fat per ¼ cup. Also avoid the creamy cold pasta, which is usually soaked in oil and, of course, the higher-fat dressings.

Meal Three: Drop by a convenience store and grab a piece of fruit or a bag of pretzels.

Meal Four: Go Italian. Order a pasta with either marinara or wine sauce, ask for plain bread instead of garlic bread, and order a salad with your dressing on the side. If you want a pizza, ask that it come with no cheese, and add a variety of vegetable toppings for flavor. If you really want to be good, ask if they'll make the pizza crust oil-free.

Meal Five: Try a nonfat yogurt at a yogurt or ice cream shop. Try to get yogurt that is less than one gram of fat per cup.

Your Day Six Workout

Complete five Sixty-Second Workouts. Include at least one stretching workout.

Evening Pep Talk

Some of you have told me that it's hard for you to work up the courage to special order. You say that you get a little embarrassed in front of the waiter or the people you're eating with, and so you say nothing. I've seen hard-driving businessmen—tough negotiators at the conference table—turn completely passive at a restaurant table.

But I have spoken to restaurant associations around the country, and I know restaurant owners want to keep you as a customer. And if you order food to be cooked a low-fat way and it comes out too high in fat, nine times out of ten the restaurant will send the food back to be redone. The manager and waiter want to make sure that you get what you have ordered. I've even gone to major banquets where all the food is fixed the same, and I've grabbed one of the people who work there and said, "Excuse me. I'm on a special eating program. Will you help me out here?" And in the middle of those banquets, they bring me what I ask for.

Special ordering at restaurants will soon be second nature for you. But until then, one good way to beat the psychological barrier you might be feeling is to call the restaurant in advance and ask about the low-fat, nonoil dishes you could order that evening. Under the Slimdown for Life, dining in restaurants can be as much fun as ever. And what will make it especially fun for you is that you can realize how much good food you can eat and walk away from the table knowing your program hasn't been sabotaged by a high-fat meal. It's an empowering feeling to know that you control what you eat, rather than letting someone else control you.

Slimdown Tip:
Don't Forget Water

A terrific secret to a better body is getting lots of water in it, as much as eight to ten glasses of water per day. Half of your body weight is composed of water, and each day your body naturally loses up to twelve cups of water. Replacing that water and keeping it circulating through your system is a secret weapon for better health, for it helps to wash out toxic waste and helps supply oxygen and nutrients to your muscles and organs. Water is also very important for weight loss, taking up a lot of room in the stomach, which keeps excessive hunger at bay. Most significantly, if you aren't drinking enough water, your body will sometimes misinterpret its own thirst as a food craving. Experts say your "hunger pangs" are often your body's request for more water. The next time you are wanting to eat between meals, try drinking water. You may find that water is just the thing to quench your hunger as well as your thirst.

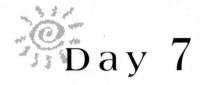

Day 7

"Active Rest"

Today you get an extra bonus—a surefire way to burn extra calories out of your fat cells. I call it "Active Rest."

One of the reasons America has gotten so much fatter over the past twenty years is that we no longer do the little day-to-day activities that are not officially considered "exercise" but go a long way in keeping us fit. Consider this report recently published on the difference between a normal working woman in 1955 versus one today. In 1955, she was likely to walk a quarter mile to the bus stop, followed by another quarter-mile walk to her job on the second or third floor of an elevatorless building. If she drove, she used a stick shift to change gears instead of an automatic transmission, which hadn't been invented yet. Because she had no electric dishwasher, she did more work in the kitchen come evening. If she watched television, she had to get up and down from her chair to change channels because there was no such thing as a remote control. And on weekends, she was far more likely to do yard work today than her 1990's counterpart, who is more likely to hire a yardman.

My point is *not* that you should give up all the conveniences in life. But by adding back into your daily routine some things that will get your body moving—by making yourself more "active" when you are at "rest"— you will be amazed at the results.

Some "Active Rest" Tips

Here are some ways to add "active rest" to your life for today:

1. Park your car at the far end of the parking lot and walk farther to your office.

2. Take a flight of stairs instead of the elevator every now and then.

3. Find ways to move around in your office. Walk to the more distant water cooler rather than the one by your desk. Walk to the corner mailbox. Pace around your office when you're thinking. At the least, don't sit for more than an hour without getting up and stretching for a few minutes.

4. If you are at home most of the day and there are stairs in your house, take a break every hour or two and climb them. Remember: As far as weight control is concerned, it's not how many flights you walk at one time, it's how many you walk over the course of the day.

5. Mow your own yard. And when you do yard work, use manual tools (hand mowers, rakes, snow shovels) instead of power tools whenever you can without exhausting yourself or risking injury.

6. When you have packages to unload from your car, take them into your house one at a time to increase the number of trips back and forth.

7. Play outside with your kids five minutes longer than usual.

8. Walk the dog.

9. Invest in a cordless phone so you can talk and walk at the same time. (Think about how many feet you could cover during a half-hour call!)

10. Give up the remote control.

Are you getting the point? I've been around a lot of people who literally spend most of their lives molding and perfecting their bodies, spending thousands upon thousands of dollars with personal trainers. But the path to good fitness hardly requires such obsession. According to the *New England Journal of Medicine,* two doctors recently determined that the average person could improve his heart as well as a die-hard fitness buff by— are you ready for this?—simply climbing stairs for six minutes a day.

Other researchers say that basic routine activity— getting up, getting dressed, lifting things, putting them down, walking around, doing housework, making business deals, going out in the evening, and so forth—will burn 25 percent of your total calories, *and that's if you are only moderately active.*

Your Day Seven Eating Guide

Meal One: If you want to try an amazing new breakfast, go for the Egg Muffin from the recipe chapter. If you eat an Egg McMuffin at McDonald's, you're getting at least 400 calories and a ton of fat. But with my Egg Muffin, you're getting a perfectly balanced, low-fat, low-calorie meal.

Meal Two: Try a delicious fat-free tuna salad. Take a can of water-packed tuna with fat-free mayonnaise. Put in diced onion, celery, and egg whites. If you wish, add Dijon mustard, vinegar, cilantro, and tomatoes. Mix it up and you have a terrific protein.

Meal Three: Run by a Chinese restaurant, and grab some steamed rice and steamed fish or chicken. (Make sure only white chicken meat is used.) Use a little teriyaki sauce for flavor.

Meal Four: Baked turkey breast, brown rice, and vegetables.

A *quick way to bake a turkey breast is to put it in a Reynolds cooking bag, add seasonings, shake it, and then bake it in the oven for twenty minutes per pound at 325 degrees.*

Meal Five: As a new evening snack, try rice cakes (which come in a variety of flavors). For a great spread, mix fat-free cream cheese and low-sugar preserves on the rice cakes. Or put fat-free cheese on top of the rice cake and melt in the oven.

Your Day Seven Workout

1. Five Sixty-Second Workouts.
2. Walk for fifteen to twenty minutes. Consciously lengthen your stride this time. The effect will be to naturally increase your energy output.

Evening Pep Talk

Can you believe that you are about to finish your first week on the program? I bet you've quickly realized that a cornerstone to your success in the Slimdown for Life is being ready for every hour of the day. If you know what you're supposed to be doing as the day unfolds, you're going to progress much more quickly than normal.

An invaluable tool for me to stay on the program is to take my daily calender and write down everything I need to do that day to guarantee that I achieve all my eating and fitness goals. It's not just a to-do list. I mark down the exact times when I should be eating my meals and what I want those meals to consist of. I mark down the times when I am going to work out and I mark down the times when I am going to take my walks. I include shopping lists for the grocery store. If I am going out to eat at night, I put down exactly what I wish to order so that I won't be tempted to order a higher-fat dish. I even write down when I'm going to pre-prepare and cook low-fat food at home. I also schedule other personal time to stay focused on my goals. In fact, on my personal calendar, I also write down ten minutes every day for what I call "Goal Time."

I highly recommend that you create a similar calendar. You might have one of those black leather personal day planners as I do, or you can use a regular spiral notebook. It doesn't matter. Just use it in order to keep yourself on track.

Merely by keeping a journal, your awareness of your habits will soar, making a huge difference in your long-term success. When you keep a written record of your eating, you'll find yourself more driven to get through a day of perfect eating. When you keep a written record of your workout times, you'll start enjoying the pattern of your workouts more; you'll hate it when you break the regularity of your workouts. Your journal will keep you moving forward, and in the Slimdown for Life, that's what counts—not postponing your program until tomorrow, not waiting to work out until "someday," but making sure success is heading your way right now!

Slimdown Tip: Don't Forget Your Fibrous Veggies

Although I have been concentrating this week on teaching you about the importance of lean proteins and starchy carbs, I don't want to de-emphasize the glory of fibrous veggies. I don't claim that you must always have them at each meal, but they are important throughout the day. High-fiber foods reduce the blood levels of insulin, a hormone that can overstimulate the appetite. High levels of fiber intake have also been associated with a decreased risk of developing heart disease, colon cancer, constipation, and diabetes. True, although starchy carbs like potatoes, beans, and rice have fiber in them, a starchy carb is more calorically dense, while a fibrous vegetable is basically water with nutrients. Whereas a cup of corn (a starchy carb) has about 150 calories, a cup of green beans (a fibrous veggie) has about 50. Fibrous vegetables can add flavor and variety to your meals and help fill you up without overloading you with calories.

Week Two

*For as long as you live, you'll have the
Slimdown for Life. There is literally
nothing that can get in your way.*

Do you realize how much is changing in you already?
You are changing just by reading about what this program involves. You are changing your habits simply by
becoming aware of what food does when it enters your
body, by realizing the advantage of burning off a few
extra calories through extra cardio activities, and by
discovering how quickly your vital lean muscle tissue
strengthens through basic Sixty-Second Workouts.

I make a point of talking to as many people as I can
who are going through the Slimdown for Life. And I've
discovered something fascinating. Those who have great
success with the Slimdown for Life are not necessarily
the ones with the most time on their hands to do extra
workouts or prepare lots of low-fat meals. They aren't
the ones with the financial resources to hire personal

trainers or pay for every new piece of fitness equipment they see on an infomercial. They aren't the stereotypical obsessive types who feel they must do anything they can to lose weight.

In truth, the most successful people on this program are the ones who relax and let the Slimdown for Life slowly and simply enhance their lives. Listen to this letter from Mary, a housewife and mother from Illinois:

Larry, I have gone through every diet you can imagine. I have starved myself more times than I want to admit. And then I heard about you. After the first week on your program, I started losing weight and I realized I hadn't starved myself once. I knew I had found my program for life.

Here's what a schoolteacher in southern California told me:

Every time I tried to go on a diet, I ended up gaining more weight. And I didn't understand why until I heard you talk. I decided to get real and get on a program that got me to lose weight naturally. You have been a godsend.

The Joys of the Journey

Let me again remind you, no matter how excited you are to change your body, this program works best only if you slowly immerse yourself into it. Yes, there have been some people on the Slimdown for Life who have lost thirty pounds in a month. But as you get into this program, I'd prefer you forget about your scales.

In fact, in the first couple of weeks of the Slimdown for Life, your clothes might start feeling loose on you, but you may not initially be losing many pounds. The reason is you'll be building sleek, lean muscle tissue as you strip away body fat—and lean muscle tissue weighs more than fat. So if you are gauging your success with your scales, you might get discouraged with me and give up and go back to a standard, old-fashioned deprivation diet.

Remember: Fad diets knock off pounds by getting rid of your water weight and your valuable muscle tissue. What counts here is permanent weight loss—the loss of fat from your body, not the speed with which you can lose ten pounds.

The Slimdown for Life is designed to change your body's metabolism and starve your fat cells—which takes more time than going on a crash-and-burn diet that you will only be able to do for a couple of weeks. The longer you go on my program, the more you'll realize that you will be able to lose as much weight as is genetically possible for your body. That's going to be a lot of weight, no matter what your genetic makeup is.

But don't be in a hurry. Relax, forget about the exact number of pounds you weigh, and concentrate on losing body fat, gaining some muscle tissue, and letting the program takes its course.

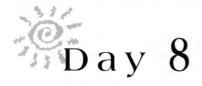

Day 8

How to Cheat

What other diet program—starts out the week by teaching you how to cheat? As perplexing as it sounds, however, part of your education in the Slimdown for Life is learning how to eat a "cheat" meal that doesn't fit the parameters of this program. I am a realist, and I know no one—not even I—can follow this program all the time. Most of us can only go so long depriving ourselves of our very favorite high-fat foods. If we feel we are being held hostage to just one particular way of eating, we will quit. With the Slimdown for Life, you are getting the best of both worlds—you will get a few cheat meals, and you will still lose weight.

If you go on a traditional deprviation diet, a cheat meal can be disastrous, adding back nearly all the weight you've lost. Why? Because your body is in such a state of starvation during your diet that the food from your cheat meal would be immediately soaked up by the fat cells like water soaking into a sponge.

In truth, the occasional cheat meal doesn't hurt you nearly as much with the Slimdown for Life. The Slimdown for Life creates a metabolism so high that it can burn through a lot of those fat calories that come from a cheat meal. Your muscles will also be far more efficient, thus capable of taking in more calories to be burned.

Now please be sure you understand. I'm not talking here about giving yourself the opportunity to go off and gorge for hours at a pizza buffet. A cheat is not an excuse to binge. Nor am I saying that you can cheat once a day. If you try to throw in a high-fat dessert every day or wolf down a hamburger at lunch five times a week, you're not going to get lean. But you can remain successful if you say to yourself, "Okay, there is going to be one time in the next two weeks when I am going to eat a great high-fat meal. I am only going to go eat one or two higher-fat dishes that I really love, and I'm going to make sure to exhibit portion control on those dishes."

A four-year study of more than 2,000 women at the Fred Hutchinson Cancer Research Center at the University of Washington in Seattle, reveals that women who limited their fat intake to around 25 percent of calories lost their taste for fat in six months or less. By the end of the study, say the women, they actually found fatty foods unpleasant to eat.

For instance, if your idea of cheat meal is a big juicy steak and loaded baked potato, then why don't you make sure there is no bread on the table and that the salad comes with a nonfat dressing. That alone will save you a chunk of calories. Or if you want a bucket of fried chicken for your cheat meal, why don't you pick out a couple of the best breast pieces and eat those with the skin, and peel the skin off the other pieces?

Perhaps you can do even a more modified cheat meal, which is eating your usual healthy meal with a cheat item on the side, and in moderation. You could get a small cut of chicken fried steak for your entrée or a half slice of pie for dessert. For some people, a taste of "high-fat" foods is enough to give them what the diet experts call "mouth satisfaction." You can then return home feeling as though you did indeed have a special night, and your waistline won't have suffered a bit. And, if you do overdo it in a cheat meal, get over it quickly and get right back on the program. It's no big deal.

You'll Lose Your Desire to Cheat

If you're wondering why I'm not particularly fearful of your having cheat meals, it's because I have seen, over and over, people get on this program, scared to death they won't ever eat their favorite foods, and within a few weeks realize that they didn't want to cheat as much as perhaps they thought they did. For the first time in their lives, looking good and feeling great have become so important to them that they actually lose their taste for the fatty foods they loved.

While you may not believe such a thing will happen to you—you're perhaps thinking right now that there is no way you'll ever give up your love of cheese fries— I know it will. As you get more experience following this program, and you keep your body well nourished with the right foods, you won't feel the same cravings for the wrong ones. In fact, *you will actually get bored with fattening foods*!

Your Day Eight Eating Guide

Meal One: Try a unique breakfast combination—oatmeal with a scoop of protein powder and sprinkled with artificial sweetener. Add sliced fruit for flavor. Or add the incredible low-fat French Toast which you can find in the recipe chapter.

Meal Two: Grilled chicken breast with a cup of rice. Or take a look at the excellent Fake Fried Chicken in the recipe chapter.

Meal Three: Roast beef sandwich and baked chips.

Meal Four: It's celebration time. Your first Cheat Meal!

Meal Five: One cup of nonfat yogurt with a half-cup of raw oatmeal or cereal mixed in.

Your Day Eight Workout

1. We're boosting your workouts. Today, go for five Sixty-Second Workouts. Include a couple of the stretching exercises in today's workouts.

2. Also today, you're moving up to a thirty-minute walk. Remember, you can break this walk up into two fifteen-minute walks, or even three ten-minute walks. But walk. Use a treadmill if you wish, walk at the local mall if you don't want to be outside, or walk with a friend. There's an extra advantage to a walking partner, for it helps you judge your pace. To maintain the best fat-burning pace, you should be able to carry on a conversation the entire time you walk. You'll work up a mild sweat, which is fine. But if you can't keep a conversation going, then you're working too hard.

Evening Pep Talk

In the Slimdown for Life, working out your mind is as important as working out your body. Indeed, your mind is like any of the other muscles of the body: You must use it or "lose it." That's why, during our Evening Pep Talks this week, we are going to work on techniques to strengthen your self-confidence and determination so that you'll stay focused on achieving your goals.

So right now, I want you to repeat this sentence: *"I am the single most important thing in my life."*

It sounds a little weird, doesn't it? In order for you to be the best person you can be, however, you first and foremost have to take care of yourself. When you treat yourself as the most important person in your life, then you will start nurturing yourself with the same passion with which you nurture anything or anyone you love. I once heard someone say, "Love yourself first, and everything else falls into line."

It's true. And that is exactly what will happen to you on this program. As you go to sleep tonight, I want you to think about your body as a temple or perhaps as your very best friend. You treat it with care. You never neglect it and you never let it get into danger. You make sure it is not abused. If you make the commitment to yourself *tonight* that your body is precious, then you will never fail.

Slimdown Tip: Beware Fat-Free Food

Although I've been suggesting some fat-free alternatives for you to use in place of your usual fattening foods, fat-free products should remain a minor part of your program. You cannot rely on them to get you lean. Most fat-free products contain a very poor balance of lean protein and starchy carbs. And fat-free hardly means calorie-free. The calories in fat-free food are the classic "empty calories" that your body sends to your fat cells. Many of you eat fat-free food all day long, believing you are doing something good for your body. But what you're doing is putting on a lot of weight because of the poor nutrition of the food. Never forget that what makes you lean is a balance of lean protein and starchy carbs. Fat-free food is merely a stopgap measure and nothing more.

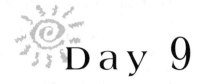

Day 9

Perfecting Your Morning Meal

Now that you've had a great cheat meal, let's get back to work. That's always the way to get back on the program after a "cheat." You never say to yourself, "Well, I might as well keep cheating for another few meals since I've already blown it today." If you overindulge, you haven't blown the program. All you have to do is pick up right back where you left off.

In many ways, the old saying is true that breakfast is the most important meal of the day—especially on the Slimdown for Life. If you're not willing to go for that first breakfast meal—and I know more people don't eat breakfast than do—you are not going to get lean on this program. There is a still pervasive myth that you can lose weight if you wake up hungry and then hold off eating until lunch. That's just not true. You've got to start feeding your body early—and you've got to feed it a balanced combination of foods. If you miss that first meal, you are undereating, and as I've told you, undereating always leads to overeating—which usually happens right at lunch.

Of course, there are those who do like to eat breakfast, but it's either a massive fat-laden meal, which is always easy to choose at breakfast (eggs, bacon, hash browns, toast with butter or pancakes with syrup, and a big glass of orange juice), or it's a very unbalanced one, like an all-carbohydrate, sugary muffin or a couple of pieces of fruit or a bowl of sugary cereal with milk. Those kinds of meals cause great fluctuations in your blood sugar levels, which then cause you to have cravings, almost always for fat or sugar.

If you are the type who loves to order the big eggs-and-bacon extravaganza, just remember that one of those breakfasts contains more than 1,000 calories, half of which are fat calories. (Again, I'm not asking you to count calories, but just keep in my mind that an average meal should be about 300–500 calories, depending on your size and whether you are male or female.) You might be thinking, "Hey, but I can work off a big breakfast all through the day—doing housework, sales calls, whatever." Sorry, that's a big myth. Remember the science: If you overload your body with calories, no matter what time of the day it is, those excess calories will head to your fat cells.

How to Eat in the Mornings

One of the biggest complaints I hear from people who don't know my program is, "Larry, I'm not sure I'm right for the Slimdown for Life because I don't like to eat egg whites, which I always hear you suggesting." I will say this until I'm blue in the face: If you hate a certain food that I suggest in your daily Eating Guide, you don't have to eat it. If you hate egg whites, don't eat them. There are plenty of other foods to eat. What's more, if there is a food you especially love, like bacon, then don't think you can never again eat another piece of bacon. That's ridiculous—of course you'll eat it, regardless of what anyone says.

All I want you to do is come up with a few ways not to rely on the fattier foods as much as you have in the past. I want you to have days where you cut down from three pieces of bacon to one piece. Or mix egg whites with whole eggs to remove a few fat calories. Substitute low-fat Canadian bacon or fat-free ham instead of regular bacon. And there are terrific low-fat morning meals, such as the Cheese Grits and Egg Muffins offered in the recipe chapter.

I recognize that you might not always get in the perfect protein–starchy carb balance in Meal One—it is sometimes very difficult to get that protein—but it is important at least to get a protein in one of your first couple of meals. Whenever you get a good protein–starchy carb meal at the very start of the morning, you've set up your body to get leaner and leaner as the day goes on. Without enough protein early in the day, your body will experience protein shortages, which will cause your blood sugar levels to fluctuate, which will then lead you to experience often uncontrollable cravings for more fat or sugar later in the day.

Your Day Nine Eating Guide

Meal One: Four to five egg whites or try an egg substitute product like Egg Beaters® with chopped veggies and a cup of oatmeal. Just to remind you: If you don't want eggs, then pick one of the Meal One items listed throughout the other days. And for a special fully balanced meal, try the Power Muffins that are listed in the recipe chapter.

Meal Two: A bowl of low-fat vegetarian chili (it can be bought at any grocery store). Add cooked ground turkey breast and beans.

My Special Fries After microwaving, boiling, or baking a potato, shave the potato into thin pieces. Cover a cookie sheet with foil and lay out the pieces. After putting the potato slices on the foil, sprinkle with spices like garlic powder, paprika, salt, and pepper. Put the potato slices in the oven and broil until brown and puffy. Flip them over with a spatula. Broil some more. Pull out the sheet and you have perfect, nonfat fries.

Meal Three: Turkey sandwich with mustard with steamed broccoli and my Special Fries.

Meal Four: Four pieces of shrimp (grilled or boiled) and one California roll sushi.

Meal Five: One grilled chicken breast, one medium-sized sweet potato with a butter substitute like Butter Buds®, and steamed veggies. One of the easiest chicken dishes is Leslie's Easy Chicken, found in the recipe chapter.

Your Day Nine Workout

1. Five Sixty-Second Workouts.
2. For extra credit, try to do three Active Rest exercises. Either get in some yard work, clean your living room windows, or walk around the house while you talk on the phone.

Evening Pep Talk

Tonight, we're going to talk about another way to keep your mind focused on your goals. Do you remember when you were a kid and you cut out magazine photographs or bought posters of your heroes and heroines? Although you didn't know it, what you were doing was envisioning a future for yourself. You were giving yourself an image of what you'd like to be. You can do the same thing in this program. I have suggested to people that they cut out a photo of someone whose body they admire. I'm not saying to find a photo of the perfect beach babe or Hollywood stud. Just get a photo of an attractive person who obviously takes care of himself or herself.

Will the picture itself give you a better body? Of course not. But it will give you a focus. Seeing someone else who has done the things you dream about can be a great inspiration for you. You could put the picture on your refrigerator and stare at it every morning as a way of helping to put in the forefront of your brain a mental image of what you want to be

This process is called "visualization." Another way to do this is to write down on a sheet of paper an image of yourself with a great body. Write down the way you think you'll look and what kind of clothes you'll be wearing. Write down the way you notice other people admiring you for the effort you made to change your body. Write down the positive, confident feelings you know you would gain if you had that better body.

By visualizing this image of yourself, over and over, you are doing nothing less than reprogramming your mind. You are imprinting upon your subconscious the fact that you are someone who is going to achieve whatever it is you set out to achieve. You will turn your dream into a reality.

Slimdown Tip: Stay Away from Fat-Burning Powders

At every health food store are products that advertise themselves as "fat burners." The products are a form of powder or juice that are supposed to help you burn off fat and increase your energy. Some products even boast they can absorb fat. But read the fine print. At most, they absorb three grams of fat—that's about the amount in half an eyedropper. Compared to a high-fat meal where you get sixty grams of fat, the benefit is tiny. The other fat-burning products are filled with additives that might have some slight impact on how lean you are. But the only ones who'll see the results from the products are those who are already extremely lean with little body fat. And in the end, you'll never be sure what you're getting. One organization studied 300 of these products and found nearly a fourth of them had no fat-burning ingredients whatsoever. Moreover, they caused such side effects as high blood pressure and heart palpitations. So why chance it for so little reward?

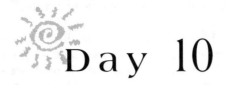

Day 10

Perfecting Your Afternoon and Evening Meals

You've probably noticed this week that I have been turning Meal Three, which last week was just a healthful snack, into a mandatory protein–starchy carb meal. Does it feel a little uncomfortable for you to imagine eating such a meal every day for the rest of your life? Generally, Meal Three falls right in the middle of the afternoon, when you are at your office or carpooling or doing just about anything except thinking about having to sit down to eat. It's one thing, you are thinking, to have a snack in the midafternoon. It's another thing entirely, you think, to have a protein–carb meal.

That's where you are wrong. In just a week and a half, you already have been given a variety of meals that you could prepare or order, from salads to sandwiches to complete dinners. You have learned about the advantage of pre-preparing meals. You've learned about meal replacement products, which you can use on occasion for Meal Three. You can use a Lean Cuisine® or Healthy Choice® entrée, both of which are not high enough in protein but will do in a pinch. You can even jump into a grocery store and grab some deli turkey or a can of white meat tuna, along with a can of corn or a baked potato from the store's deli.

No, as I've said, this is not the kind of meal that is

going to make Julia Child salivate. But neither were the snacks you were eating. The time has come for you to turn that snack into a meal because the benefits are so valuable. The person who learns to feed his body most efficiently by eating the most complete meal is the person who loses weight the fastest. As long as those meals are coming at the right intervals and in the right proportions, that food will slide right past your fat cells and head to your muscle tissue.

And Don't Forget Meal Five

The time has come for you to do something else. You must also begin treating your last evening meal, Meal Five, as a protein–starchy carb meal. One of the great misconceptions about eating is that, if you eat late at night, you will get fat. Well, if you eat what most people eat late at night—drive-through fast food or a kind of Dagwood Bumstead sandwich or ice cream and chocolate chip cookies—you will get fat. But when you eat a muscle building meal that speeds metabolism, you will get lean no matter what time it is.

A well-balanced Meal Five also keeps you from a fatty nighttime binge, and I'm sure I don't have to tell you how uncontrollable a late-night binge can be if you haven't gotten in all your meals throughout the day. I've heard dozens of stories of people who will go through the entire kitchen looking for everything sweet. Why are they doing that? Their bodies didn't get the proper balance of foods during the day. A last well-balanced meal goes a long way in keeping those fat cells quiet. One thing to be wary of during this meal, however: If you've lost a lot of fluid during the day, you'll also be tempted to pour yourself a big glass of orange juice or a soda late at night. Don't do it. Caloric beverages at night can be devastating to your body. If you're thirsty, make sure you drink lots of water late at night along with Meal Five.

Your Day Ten Eating Guide

Meal One: A one-minute breakfast of one cup of nonfat yogurt, one cup of cereal, one cup of protein powder with an artifical sweetener, and some raisins sprinkled on top.

Meal Two: Try the Apricot Chicken from the recipe chapter. Add a small dinner salad with fat-free dressing and one cup of rice and beans.

Meal Three: Try the Pizza Casserole from the recipe chapter.

Meal Four: One grilled pork tenderloin, mashed potatoes (no milk or butter), and string beans.

Meal Five: Meal replacement drink.

Your Day Ten Workout

1. It's time to push our Sixty-Second Workouts. From now on, we'll progressively increase them. Today, do eight Sixty-Second Workouts. Don't panic. You can do one workout each hour if you wish. But try to do two or three in a row so that your muscles will get a sustained workout.

2. Complete thirty minutes of walking.

The Evening Pep Talk

How's your confidence level today? One of the best ways to build your confidence and stay focused in this program is to surround yourself with like-minded people. Just one good friend can make the difference. This is someone who also might be trying to lose weight and will go through the program with you, or someone who already has been doing the program and can talk to you during those times when the desire to backslide rears its ugly head.

Ironically, some of the people you love the most or whom you perceive as your closest friends can often turn out to be your worst enemies when it comes to losing weight. They will often do some subtle and perhaps not-so-conscious things to discourage you from losing weight.

They might be well intentioned, but they could very well provide you with negative reinforcement. "Uh-oh, how long will *this* program last?" they'll wisecrack. "Are you going to last three days on this program? Maybe stretch it and go four days?"

If you have friends who are also overweight but aren't doing anything about it—which means they are probably feeling guilty about their lack of action—they might tell you, "Well, you don't look like you've lost any weight," or "You know everyone loves you for who you are, not for how you look."

You have to realize that others might feel threatened or jealous by your commitment and may try to make you feel inadequate. There will be someone going to lunch with you who will ask that you have a dessert. When you say no, he or she will inevitably say, "Oh, come on, it won't hurt you. Just eat less tonight at dinner." When you really start getting successful in this program, you are likely to hear such lines as, "I hate all this low-fat stuff you're cooking now." Or, "Aren't you embarrassed to take food with you to work?" "Please, you're not going to put us through that special ordering, are you?" "You're not going to do any Sixty-Second Workouts while we have company, are you?"

Not only do such comments hurt your feelings, they can undermine your confidence. I don't mean to be hard on you when I say this. I know it's extremely difficult to withstand social pressure. But you have to elevate yourself above people whose primary way of feeling good about themselves is to see others *not* succeed.

Never, ever be embarrassed about your desire to lose weight, and never apologize to anyone about your goals. Don't let anyone stand in the way of your decision to go after what you want! It is not egotistical or selfish to put yourself first when it comes to losing weight. You'll find a great empowerment when you start saying to others, "I want to go to a different restaurant because it's got better food for my program." You'll understand how wonderful it is to stand up for yourself when you politely say to a waiter, "This fish is swimming in oil. Could you please take it back?"

And in time, your newfound confidence will have a marvelous effect on those around you. They'll see how happy you are, how proud you've become—and soon they'll want to do exactly what you're doing, too.

Slimdown Tip: Stay Away from Candy

Are you thinking, "Well, Larry, we all know candy isn't good for you." Actually, many of you still believe that some sort of candy is a great way to get an instant burst of energy when you're feeling tired. This is a big-time fallacy. A single candy bar contains far more sugar than you need in a day, and the sugar from that candy bar sets off a major chemical imbalance in your body that, in the end, will cause you to get fatter.

Because that one candy bar causes your blood sugar levels to rise to astonishing heights, your pancreas reacts by producing an excess of insulin to deal with all that sugar. The result? The sugar from the candy bar initially makes your spirits soar, then the large dose of insulin depresses the level of blood sugar and your body suddenly slows down, causing you to feel moody, irritable, and tired—and ultimately hungrier. And what happens next? According to studies, you tend to eat a second candy bar, thinking the first one didn't do its job. And the cycle goes on and on and on. When I feel plagued by a low energy level, the one thing I like to do is take a walk. It not only gets my heart pounding, but helps release more endorphins in my brain, making me think more clearly and effectively.

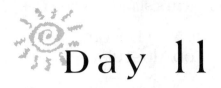# Day 11

Improving Your Workouts

I have been increasing the level of your workouts this week. Why? If you build an exercise program for yourself and then stay with that program on a regular basis, your body will learn to utilize that stored fat more quickly than it does now.

Don't forget what is happening with these extra workouts. The longer you keep your body in motion, the more your metabolism is stoked. Indeed, as you now start walking thirty minutes a day, at least four times a week, your metabolic rate will get to the point that you will continue to burn off calories at a high rate *for up to two hours after your walk.* There have been some studies that even show that on the morning after a good exercise session, a person's metabolic rate measures nearly a 5 percent increase—and that's after that person has had an eight-hour sleep!

It's also important that you increase the number of your Sixty-Second Workouts this week. You not only will be adding sleek muscle tissue that will help give your body a better shape, but are installing a fail-proof mechanism to make your weight loss much easier. You have more than four hundred muscles inside your body, each one composed of millions of tiny cells—and if you can get that muscle tissue in tip-top working shape, your body will burn calories at an enormously fast rate.

Will You Become
Too Muscular?

Let me stop and tell you that I know you are wondering, as you see the increased number of Sixty-Second Workouts, whether you should be concerned about becoming too muscular. Not in the least. Do you know what causes that overbloated look on weightlifters at gyms? They're eating too much fat. Muscle-building exercises don't make you fat; they make you lean. Muscle is to your body what gold is to the economy—the basic foundation and dynamic source of energy. In fact, simply by firming you up, the Sixty-Second Workouts can make you drop down a dress size without a major change on the bathroom scale.

And don't worry about using dumbbells in the upcoming days with your Sixty-Second Workouts. That's still not the kind of workouts that can make you, in weightlifter's parlance, "look huge." Combined with your eating program, the muscle-building exercises in this program knock out the heaviness around your hips and thighs. You get nicer, more shapely legs, and your love handles melt away. Believe me, these exercises are a lot less painful and certainly less expensive than plastic surgery.

I admit, I have stolen a few pages from bodybuilders' handbooks. Whether you love them or hate them, bodybuilders have attained a muscular development and a body fat level that was unheard of several years ago. But in the Slimdown for Life, you are never going to "get huge," to use the bodybuilder's lingo. You are not going to build bulging muscles. Nor will you ever get sore. Instead of trying to lift as much as you can, you are doing deliberate and controlled movements, focusing on the muscles you're supposed to be working.

So enjoy yourself. Every time you perform a Sixty-Second Workout, you are taking another step toward rediscovering your sexier curves and muscles.

Your Day Eleven Eating Guide

Meal One: Try the Power Muffins from the recipe chapter. Or go with egg whites, one banana, and oatmeal porridge.

Meal Two: One grilled chicken breast or turkey tenderloin with one cup of black-eyed peas. Or there's nothing better from the recipe chapter than the Taco Salad—a perfectly balanced meal in itself.

Meal Three: Here's a great, five-minute, low-fat meal. Buy a white filleted fish, rinse it, sprinkle lemon pepper over it, and squeeze half a lemon on top. Place the fish on a plate, cover in plastic wrap, and microwave for a couple of minutes. Add rice that you can boil in a bag.

Meal Four: Try the Most Requested Meat Loaf from the recipe chapter along with potatoes and green beans. If the sweet tooth is hitting you, try a soft drink float made with nonfat, low-sugar ice cream or sorbet and diet soda. Compared to more than 700 calories from a regular soft drink float, it contains a mere fraction.

Meal Five: Try the Taco Casserole from the recipe chapter.

Your Day Eleven Workout

1. Perform nine Sixty-Second Workouts.
2. For extra credit, do another walk. Try to walk this day in a hilly area. You decide the amount of time.

Evening Pep Talk

Do you remember a couple of days ago when I had you state, "I am the most important thing in my life"? Perhaps you thought I was having you do that only for dramatic effect. What you were doing, however, was called an "affirmation," and affirmations are very valuable tools. Despite their simplicity, affirmations can help drive home your belief in your own abilities.

For centuries, people have known the power of affirmations. According to ancient Hindu tradition, once we state something over and over, it becomes a "mantra," a frequently repeated thought that molds and shapes our future. The theory is that when you make an affirmation out loud, your statements are getting to your subconscious mind and transforming it so that it wills it to work to bring out the best in you. On the other hand, if we focus on our fears and insecurities, what we are really doing is inputting very negative information into our subconscious. Tell me, would you rather have a subconscious that is working against you, or one working for you?

Right now, as you're reading this, stop for just a moment and smile. Take a deep, relaxing breath and just smile. Notice how the smile changes your whole state of being. Now say, "I love improving my body."

Say it again:

"I love improving my body . . . I love improving my body."

I know, I know, it sounds silly. At least it does right

now. But you're working on your subconscious and throwing off the shackles of your old limited thinking patterns. Scientists say that on a typical day, the average person thinks about 60,000 thoughts. Even more startling is the fact that 95 percent of those thoughts are the same as the ones you had the day before. Through affirmations, you are able to install new, more empowering thoughts. Your mind has a vast, immeasurable potential that often remains untapped.

> *Feel free to create your own affirmation. Choose something that has special meaning to you.*

Your affirmations don't have to be fancy, long, or drawn-out. Here are some more you might want to say before you go to bed tonight:

"I am more fit today than ever before and I am getting fitter by the moment."

"I am growing more radiant and healthy every day."

"I'm happier and my body is growing stronger."

"Every step I'm making is progress."

"Whatever I do today, I am able to do a little bit more tomorrow."

"Whenever I eat a perfect meal, I am supercharging my body."

"Whenever I work out, I am burning off hundreds of calories."

"Every day, in every way, I am getting better, better and better."

Like many of you, I once thought affirmations were sort of goofy. But as I've learned, the more positive thoughts I have had about my body, the easier it has been for me to stay lean. By saying out loud what it is you want, you will give credibility to what you are doing.

Slimdown Tip: Interval Walking

Here's a way to get an extra boost out of your walking program. Every now and then, try something called "interval walking." That's when you alternate your basic walking pace with some higher-intensity spurts. For example, first start off for ten minutes at your regular moderate rate. Then pick up the pace until you're breathing harder (but not all out) for a couple of minutes, then slow back down to your regular speed that lets you catch your breath, which will probably be slower than your initial walking speed. Then pick up the pace again for another couple of minutes, and so on, and so on.

This kind of training allows you to burn more calories per minute, and will keep you at a higher metabolic rate throughout your walk. It's going to help with the afterburn effect, too. You'll be burning fat at a higher rate even after you stop exercising. The more intense the exercise, the greater the afterburn effect.

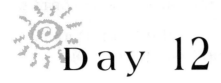

Day 12

Improving Your Protein Intake

It's usually around this period in the program when I sometimes hear people say, "Larry, I've never eaten this much protein in my life. Are you sure all the protein on your program is good for me?"

After years of misinformation about protein being harmful to your kidneys and so on, the current medical research has proven that not only is protein good for your body (including your kidneys), but many scientists are suggesting we could eat more of it. We have twenty very important amino acids in our body that help build muscle—ten of which the body sustains, and the other ten of which must be gotten from the protein we eat. So the higher the quality of protein you can get into your body, the better off you'll be.

While it might appear that I'm encouraging you to eat a lot of protein on this program, the truth is that you have probably been very deficient in the past in getting the right kind of protein into your body. And remember, you're not eating that much protein. Ten egg whites might seem like a lot of food. But it has the same number of calories as two whole eggs with a lot less fat. A five-ounce grilled chicken breast seems like a lot of food, but it has the same number of calories as half a candy bar.

Improving the Beef, Poultry, and Fish in Your Diet

In recent years, meat producers have adopted new breeding and feeding methods that have reduced the fat content of their animals. Even so, beef is still a major source of fat in the American diet. In general, you should eat beef less frequently, and even then only with care—for even when beef appears lean, it still has more than 30 percent fat. Let me repeat myself from early on in the book: Cuts such as tip round, top round, and top sirloin have less fat than other cuts. When choosing those cuts, look for the ones that have the least amount of visible fat or marbling throughout the muscle. The longer you cook it, the more fat that will be burned off. The fattiest cuts include ribs and tenderloin. And stay away from liver, kidney, heart, and tongue, except on rare occasions. Finally, keep your portion sizes very, very small. I recommend about three or four ounces per serving. That's a portion that is approximately the size of a deck of playing cards.

I must admit that, as much as I love a good steak, I tend to go with poultry or fish on this program. In many cases, it provides a higher-quality protein, and most important, it is lower in total fat than beef. In seafood such as cod, haddock, and yellow-fin tuna, the fat content is incredibly low. Haddock, for instance, gets about 8 percent of its calories from fat in a typical serving. And even the higher-fat, dark-meat fishes such as salmon give you a less saturated fat than beef.

Always go for white meat in chicken and turkey. Dark meat can be as high in fat as beef. And always go for skinless white meat. Dark skinless chicken meat contains about 8.3 grams of total fat in a typical three-ounce cooked serving; 43 percent of its calories come from fat. But white skinless chicken breast contains 3.8 grams of fat in a typical three-ounce serving; only 23 percent of the calories come from fat. And listen to this: If you leave the skin on that chicken breast, the number of calories from fat doubles.

Your Day Twelve Eating Guide

Meal One: Try egg whites along with the Cheese Grits dish you will find in the recipe chapter.

Meal Two: Large salad with grilled chicken and nonfat dressing. You can add corn to your salad for your starchy carb. If you're adventurous, try the Chicken Broccoli Rice Casserole from the recipe chapter.

Meal Three: Turkey sandwich, baked potato, and steamed veggie.

Meal Four: Try one of the pizzas in the recipe chapter.

Meal Five: Try the Rio Grande Chicken Stew in the recipe chapter.

Your Day Twelve Slimdown Workout

1. Perform ten Sixty-Second Workouts. This is the most we'll go for the week. Schedule them into your daily calendar so that you are certain you will get them all in.

2. Another mandatory walk: thirty minutes.

Evening Pep Talk

You've already learned to do several things in the Pep Talks this week to build a more powerful attitude—visualizing yourself at your best and using affirmations to stay motivated. Tonight, I want you to work on pushing negative thoughts out of your mind altogether.

Can you imagine going for the rest of the night without thinking a single negative thought? Can you do that? Spend the next two or three hours with a 100 percent positive mental attitude? That is what truly confident and successful people do. They can turn their backs on negative situations by saying, "Don't give it another thought." They specialize in putting positive thoughts into their minds—and keeping them there.

Try this. Take a few moments tonight and recall some pleasant, positive experiences. Count your blessings. Recall the many good things you have to be thankful for: your spouse, your children, your friends, your health. Recall the good things you saw people do today. Recall your little victories and accomplishments. Go over the reasons why you are glad to be alive. You might write all these thoughts down on a sheet of paper.

Then conscientiously visualize yourself putting those thoughts into what I like to call your "memory bank." In time, those thoughts, as you dwell on them, become the dominant thoughts in your memory bank. The negative thoughts have more trouble taking up space in your brain and trying to draw you off course.

Psychologists say that what you are doing is reconditioning your mind. You are developing a mode of thinking without limitations. By pushing a positive attitude on yourself, you are not trying to look unrealistically at life through rose-colored glasses. Rather, you are celebrating the wonders of life. You are seeing the cup as half full rather than half empty.

Remember, winners are always looking for opportunities. They deal with problems as soon as they arise. Instead of focusing on the breakdowns, they move forward by focusing on finding solutions—right now!—with zest and drive.

Slimdown Tip: Vary Your Cardio Routine

One of the best ways to boost your walking program is to take your act on the road. Find new parks or neighborhoods. Take walking vacations in other cities. Just to see how you feel about it, go to your local gym—you can usually pay a daily fee without having to join—and do nothing but walk on the treadmill for thirty minutes. Time flies when you're on a treadmill and you get to watch everyone else around you working out.

And just to remind you about something I said a while back: If you get tired of walking, you can do something else for the cardio phase of your program. You can attend a dance class. Rent an exercise tape from your video store. You can jog. Run long distances. Ride your bike or even buy a stationary bicycle. Rollerblading is amazingly effective, as are stair climbers at gyms. I know people who have cross-country ski simulation machines in their homes, and I know people who swim an hour a day. If you keep variety in your program, you'll never get bored.

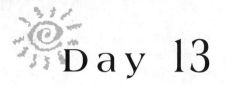

Day 13

Cutting Back Flour-Based Products

Today, we get to one of the little-understood enemies that keep you from getting lean—flour-based products like bagels, bread, pastas, and cereals.

Since such foods are technically carbohydrates—as well as being nutritious and low in fat—you might think that I would want you to eat them. I agree, these foods can be good for you—*if you eat them in much smaller amounts than you're accustomed to!* But I don't consider these flour-based products to be the kind of carbs that should be a staple of your program.

The reason they can be harmful is because of how they are made. These carbs have been altered from their natural wheat state and turned into calorie-packed "processed" food. When the natural wheat grain has been mashed and broken down into a simple flour, it is very easy for your body to digest. Because the body doesn't have to do anything to break down that processed flour-based food, the calories almost go straight into your bloodstream and then right to your fat cells.

Let me give you an example. One large-sized bagel that you see at a bagel shop has more calories than a chicken breast and a baked potato.

Let me give you an idea about cereal. All your life you've been told that nut-and-grain cereal is good for you. It is, to some extent. But one serving, which amounts to 450–500 calories, is just *three tablespoons*— or about one shot glass. In my program, you could get the same number of calories by eating twenty egg whites, two cups of oatmeal, and three slices of dried toast.

So you've got to be extremely careful of foods made of processed flour. I see people throwing down two or three bagels in the morning and thinking they're doing something healthful for themselves. They just couldn't be more wrong. The way to eat processed flour foods is in moderate portions.

On the Other Hand, Beware the Lure of Low-Carb Diets

There are many so-called "experts" who have been receiving a lot of attention recently because of their promotion of a very old concept: the low-carb, high-fat diet. The theory behind these diets is that without any carbohydrates for energy, the body will turn much more quickly to stored fat. Furthermore, say the low-carb, high-fat advocates, if you eat extra dietary fat in the process, you'll feel full longer, which means you won't eat as much. Somehow, the advocates tell you, the extra fat you're eating won't really affect your weight all that much. So in the latest rash of trendy best-selling books, what you are being given are recipes that, according to a study by the American Dietetic Assocation, contain anywhere from 41 percent to 85 percent fat. (Remember, I suggest that your foods contain only 20 percent fat.)

Yes, it is true, if you suddenly deprive your body of all carbohydrates, you'll lose weight quickly. But you're not losing body fat, and the weight you are losing is water weight, which is not going to stay off for very long. You can't possibly exist in such a nutritionally unbalanced and unhealthy state for the rest of your life. Sending your body into some unnatural carbohydrate-less state will leave you feeling tired and irritable, it will leave you without any energy, and it will make you more prone to disease, especially if you follow these diets and start eating so much fat, which is exactly what leads to heart disease and some forms of cancer. What these books also forget to tell you is that the no-carboydrate diets might eventually lead your body into a condition called "ketosis," which is a nutritional disease that can ultimately cause liver and kidney damage.

I hate to be coarse, but the new low-carb diets that are getting publicized are garbage! The reason we are fat is because we're eating too much fattening food! Carrots, rice, potatoes, and proper amounts of pasta don't get you fat. Fast food, fried food, cake, candies and the like get you fat.

Your Day Thirteen Eating Guide

Meal One: Veggie omelette made with four to six egg whites and one cup of grits with Butter Buds®.

Meal Two: Meal replacement drink.

Meal Three: Try the Shrimp Scampi from the recipe chapter.

Meal Four: Grilled venison or lean beef, mashed potatoes, and a dinner salad.

Meal Five: How about one of the lean ground beef burgers from the recipe chapter?

Your Day Thirteen Workout

1. Ten Sixty-Second Workouts.
2. You want some great extra credit? Find an office building and walk up three flights of stairs and then back down again.

Evening Pep Talk

Here's another way for you to work tonight on getting more negative thoughts out of your brain: Whenever a negative thought hits, immediately stop and try to rephrase it as a positive thought. In regard to this program, for instance, you might feel guilty (which is a negative thought) if you happen to blow your eating program one day and devour a high-fat meal. What if instead of sighing and thinking, "Wow, I was bad," you immediately imagine yourself succeeding (which is a positive thought). You imagine yourself sitting down to eat a perfect meal. You imagine the happiness you feel at eating that meal. You imagine how it's making you healthier and how it's changing your physical appearance. If you have those images in your head when you sit down at your next meal, you will eat a perfect meal.

I want you to learn to talk to yourself in a different way. It's very important that you learn to monitor the sentences that you say to yourself, replacing phrases that weaken you with phrases that empower you. That's means getting the words "can't" and "don't" out of your vocabulary. If you ever catch yourself saying or even thinking the words "bad" or "cheat" or "stupid," take a minute to change them to positive ones.

Don't say, "It's going to be difficult to cut back desserts." Say, "This is going to be an opportunity to get lean."

Don't say, "Losing weight is a struggle." Instead say, "Losing weight is a great journey."

Instead of telling yourself, "I was bad to have that piece of cake," say, "I did eat that cake, and I will be more careful at my next meal."

Instead of saying, "I must deprive myself of lots of food to lose weight," rechannel those negative thoughts into a more positive and accurate attitude. When you face a difficult situation, say to yourself, "I'll win," not "I might lose." When opportunity appears, think "I can do it," never "I can't."

In other words, let all variations of the thought "I will succeed" dominate your thinking process. When you constantly worry about getting fat (a negative thought), you are actually programming your subconscious to stay overweight because you're letting the fear of fat overwhelm you. When you stare at yourself in the mirror and say, "Gosh, it's going to take a long time to lose weight" (a negative thought), you are already trying to rationalize failure—which means you are more likely to fail. You are more likely to succeed if your brain is being given thoughts that success is the only option.

The important thing to remember is that you can find ways to break up the negative voice inside you. You can interrupt that voice, and then destroy it. No one is forcing you to listen to your negative voice. You can turn it off whenever you wish. And it is at that very moment when you really start doing your best.

Slimdown Tip: Buy Dumbbells

As your workouts are progressing, it is probably time for some—though not all—of you to start holding light dumbbells in your hands during your Sixty-Second Workouts. They cost around 39 cents a pound and they can be purchased at any sporting goods or fitness store. A set of two-, three-, five-, eight-, and ten-pound dumbbells—ten total—will probably cost you $25. Or, if you want to economize, try using one gallon jugs of water. You'll be amazed at the results. If you have been following the workouts, your body has begun to quickly recondition itself, and if you want to improve on that level of fitness, you need to add some resistance. You are ready to move to the next step in which your muscles begin to reshape your body in a stunning, beautiful way. With less fat on your body, you'll really see more results in a hurry. But again, you don't have to do it. You'll get great results if you just stay with weightless workouts.

Day 14

Dealing with Snacks

Even though you are now eating five times a day—and you are trying to include a lean protein and starchy carb in as many of those meals as possible—there will still be times when many of you are going to find yourself wanting to nibble between meals. Some of you might be able to wait every three hours for your next meal. For others of you, the urge to eat will sometimes show up an hour and a half after a meal, and you decide you absolutely have to snack before the next meal.

I'm going to be honest with you. Snacking can counteract all the benefits of the program, and on occasion it can sabotage the Slimdown for Life. I know people who oversnack on high-fat food and then say to themselves, "Well, I've blown it now. I might as well blow the rest of the day, too." They are like dominoes: Once the first bit of control goes, the rest follows, and soon their whole eating program collapses.

If done correctly, however, snacking can enhance your program. You can allow snacking to play a role in your life, but I'm warning you, you have to be very, very careful. For many of us, the kinds of snacks we turn to are the very foods that can "trigger" a reaction in us to splurge. You might think, "Oh, I'll have just one cookie," and then boom! You've had four or five. Or how many of you have walked through the kitchen and grabbed a handful of potato chips, thinking it's perfectly okay to have just three or four chips—and then fifteen minutes later you grab another handful on your next trip through the kitchen?

Or how many of you have eaten a spoonful of ice cream on one trip to the kitchen, then some fried tortilla chips on another, then a few allegedly low-fat cookies on another trip, and then a slice of cold pizza on another trip? You might laugh, but I know lots of people who constantly graze through their refrigerators in between meals and still believe they are following the program.

Many snack foods are called "trigger foods" by nutritionists because they are the ones that you can't "have just one" of once you've started. They are the foods that prompt chain eating, and they can be just as difficult to kick as chain smoking.

Now I have said many times in this book that you can do this program without having to give up your favorite foods. But right now, you need to have a big talk with yourself. If you are one who gets really hungry while doing this program, will you be able to snack successfully as long as there are plenty of salty, high-fat foods or desserts in the kitchen?

I told you already that I have banned peanut butter from my house. I also have done the same thing with ice cream and pies and sugary cereals and other processed foods loaded with fat calories. For me, there can be no equivocation with trigger foods. If I think a specific food has a certain temptation for me, and it can affect the quality of my program, that food has to go.

You don't have to go that far, of course. You don't have to do the program as strictly as someone like me. On the other hand, try to have your kitchen stocked with low-fat snacks. I am big on eating fibrous vegetables for snacks. They fill me up without giving me any fat calories. I will down a green salad or eat a bag of cut-up carrots, celery, or broccoli. I'll eat an apple, which at sixty calories is just fine. (Remember my earlier warning: If you eat more than a couple of pieces of fruit, you're overloading your body with lots of simple carbohydrates, which are easy to digest and can easily be picked up by your fat cells.)

New Snacks for Your Program

If you're going to eat between meals, then having the right kind of snacks in your house becomes absolutely critical to losing weight. If you're willing to throw out all your greasier salty snacks and your sugary desserts, then try these:

1. Fresh fruit, dill pickles, and fresh vegetables.
2. Fat-free chips and crackers, rice cakes, and low-fat pretzels. Use them with dips such as picante sauce, picante sauce mixed with fat-free cream cheese, picante sauce mixed with fat-free dressing, or fat-free spinach dip.
3. Air-popped popcorn. (Try *lightly* spraying the popped corn with butter-flavored cooking spray, then sprinkle with cajun seasoning, chili powder, or fat-free cheese.)

4. Fat-free yogurts, low-calorie Popsicles, and artificially sweetened puddings.

5. Low-fat vegetable soup.

6. A cheeseless pizza.

Your Day Fourteen Eating Guide

Meal One: Low-fat Egg Muffin, from the recipe chapter, with baked hash browns purchased from the frozen foods section of your grocery store.

Meal Two: Four to five ounces of baked turkey breast, steamed vegetable, and one cup of bean and corn salad.

Meal Three: Baked fish and, for your carb, try the Rice Salad from the recipe chapter.

Meal Four: Try the Pasta with Ham and Peas from the recipe chapter.

Meal Five: Meal replacement drink or a low-fat frozen meal.

Your Day Fourteen Workout

1. Ten Sixty-Second Workouts.

2. Thirty minutes of walking.

4. End-of-the-week bonus: Do extra stomach crunches. One of the great myths of fitness is that if you do more sit-ups, your stomach gets smaller. Not true: Only proper eating can take care of that. But I've discovered if you do enough crunches until you feel a tightening of stomach muscles through the rest of the

day, you'll be far more aware of what you eat to keep your stomach from getting bigger!

Evening Pep Talk

Did you feel completely refreshed as you went through the day today? If so, I bet it had a lot to do with what you have been doing to your mind this week. By trying to rid yourself of negative thoughts, by going to bed thinking only of positive things about yourself, you unknowingly gave your subconscious a chance to exhale. Instead of being burdened with a lot of depressing junk, your subconscious was able to luxuriate in more creative, nourishing thoughts.

There's no way around it: The more positive thoughts you have about yourself, the more you will base your decisions upon those positive thoughts. The more you say to yourself, "I can succeed on the Slimdown for Life," the more you are guaranteeing success. When you say to yourself affirmations such as "I am the most important person in my life," or "I deserve to do something good for myself," then good things will happen. Without that jolt of self-esteem—without that fervent belief in your own value—you will allow yourself to stay stagnant. You will think you are too old or too out-of-shape or too busy or too whatever to get the body you want.

As Confucius said many years ago, "Good people can strengthen themselves ceaselessly." And that's exactly what you're doing.

Congratulations. It's on to Week Three.

6

Week Three

The amazing thing about this program is that you don't merely renew your body—you also renew your mind.

I cannot tell you how much I love meeting people who have finished the second week of the Slimdown for Life. It's not just the obvious physical progress that I've seen—the change in shape of their bodies—but it's seeing in their eyes the realization that they are on their way to true, unqualified success. After I gave a speech one day to a group about the Slimdown for Life, Trish, a secretary from Dallas, approached me and said, "Larry, when I first heard about you, I didn't really trust you. I didn't think you were shooting straight with us. But I decided to go ahead and follow your program—at least for a few days."

"What happened?" I asked.

"By the second week, I felt a sense of energy I never had before. I felt really, really healthy! I was eating the right kind of foods, and I was eating a lot of them. But . . ."

"But what?"

"I still didn't think I was going to lose weight."

"Well, what happened then?"

Trish smiled. "Over the next three months, I lost twenty-five pounds—and I could tell it was all body fat. I've never felt so good in my life."

Over and over, I have heard these kinds of stories— men and women who thought there was no answer for them, who thought they didn't have the willpower to lose weight, who figured they'd stay heavy for the rest of their lives—and who then discovered the Slimdown. In the process of transforming their bodies, they started transforming the power of their minds. They learned to dream again. Some began to think positive thoughts about themselves for the first time in years.

One of the most inspiring stories I ever heard came from a very down-on-his-luck, overweight man who lived in a boardinghouse. He wrote and told me that he had plugged in an old AM radio and listened to my call-in radio show as a form of entertainment. But over the months, as he kept listening to me say that people can change their entire lives just by changing their bodies, this man decided to change his body, too. He was close to homeless, and he had been eating mostly cheap processed and fried foods, foods high in salt and fat. But he bought a little hot plate, then he began buying oatmeal and rice, canned tuna and white chicken in water, and canned vegetables for his fiber. He began eating five small meals a day, the price of which he said cost him less than one meal at a fast-food outlet. He walked in a pair of old tennis shoes, averaging thirty minutes five times a week. Within three months, he later told me, his energy was up, his negative attitude was gone, and for the first time in a decade, he decided to pursue a goal for his own life. He wrote me that he had received a full-time job, found a place of his own to live, and had lost thirty pounds.

If this man could find the motivation to do this program when he was barely keeping a roof over his head, then what excuse do any of us have not to do it?

You Must Stay Alert

In our final week together, we will focus our energies on maintaining the Slimdown—staying in control and developing the right kind of coping mechanisms during those periods when we backslide and relapse into our old habits. You'll be fine-tuning your skills.

And believe me, the old habits will try to return. There will be times when you'll become so emotionally stressed out that you'll want to drown your feelings in food (the fattier the better). There will be other times when you are walking alone and you start smelling something wonderful coming from a bakery. Boom. You'll want to race inside and order everything you see.

You might be making peanut butter and jelly sandwiches for your kids, and you find yourself making little sandwiches for yourself. You might find yourself at business dinners, thinking you must eat and drink as much as your customers to make them feel comfortable, regardless how much it wrecks your program. At other times, you'll get so busy at work or with your family that you'll start missing your walks or your Sixty-Second Workouts. There will be a voice inside you trying to make you think that missing a few walks or having a few mini–peanut butter sandwiches isn't going to matter.

It's foolish to think that your healthy new habits will

hold up to your old, ingrained habits if you do not stay vigilant. There will be days when you wake up without any enthusiasm, and the last thing you want to do is pre-prepare some meals. As you start hitting your target weight, the weight won't be coming off as fast (that's because it won't need to), and you will no longer have the exhilarating reward as you once did about the fat dropping off your body.

Trust me, you will have lapses. You will make mistakes.

But here's the thing to remember: A successful person isn't someone who makes no mistakes. It's someone who knows how to deal with them when they happen. That's why our work this week can be summed up in three words: maintenance, coping, and control. We will work at maintaining our program, coping with mistakes, then getting back in control.

You're not going to avoid thinking about your setbacks. You're going to deal with them. You're no longer going to shrug guiltily and say to yourself that you need more "willpower." You're going to learn "control power" that will make eating right and staying fit as automatic and natural as breathing.

It's not always as exciting to maintain your weight as it is to lose it. But you've worked too hard to get to this point to have to start all over again. Let's truly make this time *the last time* you ever have to lose weight again.

Day 15

Separating Emotions from Food

I want us to start off this week by confronting a major enemy in our quest for leanness: the reason we over-indulge ourselves with food. How many times have you eaten a huge dinner at a restaurant and then, the minute you got home, started looking for something to eat? Although your stomach was full, something else was missing. You weren't satisfied. And for some uncon-scious reason, you decided it was more food that would help you find that satisfaction.

Studies have found that overweight people tend to overeat in response to stress. Any negative emotion—anger, depression, loneliness, boredom, or frustra-tion—triggers a bout of overeating. Even when they are not under stress, many people with weight problems use food as a mood elevator. They get fatigued or bored, they get lonely or just mildly fidgety—and they eat. Food becomes their way to get through life's ups and downs.

I'm not a psychologist, but after years of watching people struggle to get lean, I know that until you learn to separate your emotional life from your eating life, you're not going to be very successful on *any* weight loss program. If you turn to chocolate to deal with your feelings of anxiety, you're going to have a lot more difficulty following this program than someone who does not. If you're someone who can "go blank" while eating—letting your feelings disappear underneath a mound of food—you're in a very precarious, high-risk position to get even fatter.

To some degree, all of us have to break the practice of using food to get emotional satisfaction. I have gone through the same struggle myself. I grew up in a family that turned to food for solace and I know that I, too, have a tendency to be a compulsive overeater, no different from my mother or grandmother. One evening a few years ago, my wife shocked me when I came home and told her in this semiarrogant tone of voice, "Honey, isn't it great that I don't take out my frustrations at the office on you or my family?"

She said, "That's right, Larry, you take out your frustrations on the refrigerator. You come home and you don't stop eating."

It took me a while, but I later realized she was right. Although I was always eating more healthful foods, I would eat anything I could get my hands on if I had had a stressful day—an entire bag of air-popped popcorn, followed by a bag or two of baby carrots, followed by six sugar-free Popsicles—all in one sitting!

How to Stop Your Emotional Eating

I am not about to mislead you into thinking that this program is going to prevent stress and tension from entering your life. We live in the real world. And as good as you might be at this program, there will be times when you'll be caught with your guard down, when stress will rear its ugly head and you'll want to eat to swallow your negative mood.

That's why you need good solid strategies to keep your moods from determining how much you eat. Here are a few proven techniques:

1. When you're angry or upset, go out for a ten-minute walk. Such a move gets you away from food, and the exercise that comes from it will calm you. Did you know that when you exercise, your body releases endorphins that will combat stress? A ten-minute walk is a great answer.

2. When you get upset or stressed, stop and ask yourself questions. And ask them out loud for emphasis. *What has happened to upset me? How will food help me deal with this? Is it worth risking my new body in return for a few seconds of gratification through food?* By taking a breather, quieting down your mind, and asking some logical questions, you will start realizing the futility of using food for emotional relief. At the least, such a move will help you delay your first bite of food—and every minute you can delay yourself from eating will work to your advantage.

3. If you still find yourself headed toward the kitchen and you're not exactly sure why, try to stop dead in your tracks and ask yourself why you want something to eat at that very moment. Often, that moment of reflection is enough to turn you back around. Seriously, as simple as it sounds, you want to keep asking yourself questions. *Am I really hungry? Are these true hunger pangs I'm feeling? Or am I eating to fulfill some other need?* You might not have every single answer, but by taking the time to ask the questions, you will be throwing roadblocks in front of your seemingly "impulsive" need to eat.

Your Day Fifteen Eating Guide

Meal One: Meal replacement drink.

Meal Two: Scrambled egg whites with vegetables and diced baked potato.

Meal Three: Grilled chicken breast, rice, and salad.

Meal Four: Fat-free cottage cheese on toast.

Meal Five: Try the Taco Salad dish from the recipe chapter. Add a mashed potato and green beans.

Your Day Fifteen Workout

1. Ten Sixty-Second Workouts. Do four upper-body workouts, four lower-body workouts, and two stretches.
2. A thirty- to sixty-minute walk.

Evening Pep Talk

Clearly, there are ways to deal with emotional eating without spending thousands of dollars at a psychiatrist's office. Indeed, you can work some magic in your own life simply by believing the statement "I am in control." I hate to say it, but that is about as much a magic formula as I can offer. By taking control—by saying you alone and not your emotions will determine what you do— you can make your life much more special. Such control doesn't mean deprivation; it means liberation.

When I need emotional reinforcement, I make extra affirmations about myself and the benefits of this program. It keeps the negative voices from getting too loud inside me, and it keeps me focused on what I need to do. Here's a unique idea: If you own something like a Walkman, then tape-record a series of your own affirmations and play them back to yourself while you do your daily walks or complete tasks around the house. You can be as creative as you want, talking at length into the tape recorder about the joys of dropping a dress size or, for men, a smaller waist size in pants. Or you could read the following affirmation into the tape recorder:

- I am not afraid to be slender and to be healthy.
- I am open to new challenges.
- I am able and willing to commit to anything that's important to me.
- I can stay committed no matter what.
- From now on, I am committed forever to my body.
- Even if I stop, I know I can start again.
- Nothing will get in my way.

Slimdown Tip: Avoiding Sugar Cravings

Many of you think you have such a "sweet tooth" that you will still crave sugar on this program, especially at night. How can you avoid sugar "cravings" like a chocolate attack? There is an easy answer: Make sure you don't miss meals, and make sure that each meal is balanced with protein and starchy carbs. When you get a great sugar craving, it almost always means you are undereating during the day, either by missing meals or having portions that are too small. If you must address the craving, look at my suggestions for fat-free or very low-calorie desserts in the recipe chapter. These are far, far better than a sugary eating binge.

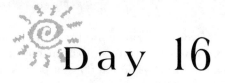

Day 16

Staying Cognizant of Your Eating

Even if you learn to recognize and control your emotional reasons for overeating, some of you might overeat for another reason. And it's the most simplistic reason you can imagine:

You'll overeat because you're used to overeating.

Now think about this. How many of you in the past two weeks have sat down to eat a meal straight from your daily Eating Guide and ended up eating far more than you'd intended to? You knew the exact portions that I wanted you to eat—your protein should be the size of your hand, your starchy carb should be about the size of your fist, and your fibrous vegetable should be able to fit into a small cereal bowl—but when you got through those portions, you kept eating.

Why did you do that? It's merely because you're just accustomed to overeating—which is not surprising considering that you have grown up in a culture that throws food at you. When the National Institutes of Health reported in 1998 that 97 million Americans were "overweight," the Institute concluded that few people knew how to stay in control around food. In other words, we would start eating and keep eating, not really giving a second thought to the fact that we were eating twice as much as we needed to.

Strategies to Keep You Cognizant

The way to start breaking the overeating habit is to follow one hard-and-fast rule: *Never let your mind wander during meals*. That's what I had to learn to do, and it helped immeasurably. I had to concentrate on what I was doing and focus on eating only the food I was supposed to eat. I firmly believe that if you can just become aware of what your eating behavior is—and if you can keep your mind alert so that it will send out warning signals the moment you start going overboard—then you'll break your overeating habits.

But how do you do that? How do you make sure that you stay focused and that you eat only the amount of food you're supposed to eat at that meal?

Try the following strategies:

1. Put your fork down between each bite. Allow a full thirty seconds to elapse between bites.

2. Never eat while standing up. Many weight-loss experts say that, if standing, you're not paying attention, and of course, if you're not paying attention to your eating, you're not in control.

3. Don't watch television or read a book or newspaper while eating. Stay focused on your meal.

4. When sitting down to a meal, don't leave serving bowls on the table. That way, you will have greater resistance to having seconds. Before you sit down for your meal, place all of your leftovers in storage containers and put them in the refrigerator.

5. Leave the table as soon as you have finished eating.

6. Put your watch or a clock in front of you and let twenty minutes elapse before you make a decision about whether to eat more. Don't forget the rule that I told you

about earlier in the book—that it takes twenty minutes for your brain to realize your body is full.

Your Day Sixteen Eating Guide

Meal One: Mix a half cup of oats and one scoop of protein powder with one cup of yogurt.

Meal Two: Meal replacement drink.

Meal Three: Eat at a Chinese restaurant. Try steamed shrimp, vegetables, rice, with garlic sauce on the side.

Meal Four: Chicken breast and baked potato with a fibrous veggie.

Meal Five: Try the Taco Casserole from the recipe chapter.

Your Day Sixteen Workout

1. Ten Sixty-Second Workouts. Do four upper-body workouts, four lower-body workouts, and two stretches.
2. For extra credit, do an "interval walk," which we talked about last week.

Evening Pep Talk

I hope before you go to bed tonight, you read these techniques again on staying focused during a meal. Perhaps right now, while you are still supercharged to do well on the program, you think you won't need them. But in the future, if you ever feel yourself slipping, these little tricks will be very important in keeping you focused—and most important, keeping you in control.

Slimdown Tip: Using Artificial Sweeteners

There was a report released a few years ago that said that aspartame, the ingredient in artificial sweeteners, could lead to brain cancer. Although the report scared everyone, it has since been thoroughly disproven as having no scientific basis. Meanwhile, there have been numerous studies conducted of aspartame, and one study in particular was conducted based on a human being using fifty times more aspartame than anyone would ever consume. It was abundantly clear that aspartame was not in any way bad as critics suggested. If you want to avoid artificial sweeteners, that's fine with me. Be sure to use aspartame in diet sodas, puddings, desserts, coffee, or tea, in moderation. However, if you feel uncomfortable using artificial sweetners, just cut down on the sugar or honey and you should be just fine.

Day 17

Eating in Social Situations

I have had so many people tell me that they do well on the Slimdown for Life when they eat alone or with a friend or supportive family member. But it's much different in social situations. At parties, they are surrounded by food—plenty of food. They find themselves standing next to tables loaded down with snacks. They sit down for a large dinner to stare at heaping plates of food. Occasionally they find themselves at dinner parties where the hostess virtually insists they eat.

What should you do? Well, clearly, there are going to be certain times—holidays, special occasions, and vacations—where it is just fine to cheat. But you don't want to feel burdened by the pressure to overeat every time you are in a social setting. You want to know for sure that you can stay in control. And wouldn't it be nice at the end of an evening not to have to make excuses to yourself about why you ate that piece of cake at the dinner party?

Learning to be a good social eater will pay off. If you're good at sticking to your program around people who want you to shed your discipline and cheat, then you'll be able to handle just about anything.

How to Face Social Pressure

If you're in a social situation, here are some ideas you can use to stay on your Slimdown.

1. Don't go to a social event on an empty stomach. It's smart to get in a well-balanced lean protein and starchy carb meal before a big event so you won't overeat the wrong foods. I even recommend that if you are going out in the evening, and you suspect you might be tempted by high-fat dishes at the restaurant you are visiting, then have a light meal beforehand. You won't be so hungry when you walk into that restaurant that you go overboard.

> Head straight for the bar and ask for a diet soda or sparkling water. It's always more difficult to eat when you have a drink in your hand.

2. Don't go for the appetizers or hors d'oeuvres at a party. It's rare to find foods like this that are low-fat. And, they are finger foods. You can throw down a dozen high-fat appetizers throughout an evening and convince yourself you're doing nothing wrong because each appetizer was so small.

3. Don't study the high-fat foods and say, "Wow, that looks so delicious." You're sending a message to your subconscious that you really want these foods, which means you'll probably eat them. Also, what you might not know is that many of our hunger impulses begin visually. They start with the eyes, not with the mouth. So in this case, out of sight is truly out of mind.

4. Take other defensive measures. Make a point of keeping a glass of seltzer water or diet soda in your hands at all times.

5. Never, ever worry about turning down someone who wants you to try something. All you need to say is, "Thanks, but I don't want any right now" (and then don't eat it later when asked again). And there's always the great health excuse: "Oh, sorry, I'm allergic to chocolate." "I'm allergic to dairy."

6. Be proud of the fact that you are different. If other people give you a kind of quizzical, slightly scornful look because you refuse food ("Oh, come on," they'll say, "one little piece isn't going to hurt you"), it's because they want to justify their own social overeating. Don't let them draw you in.

7. Enjoy the party.

Your Day Seventeen Eating Guide

Meal One: Four to six scrambled egg whites with vegetables, and one cup of creamed rice cereal.

Meal Two: Chicken breast and rice.

Meal Three: Try some sushi. Three pieces of shrimp sushi (no avocado or mayonnaise), one tuna sashimi (no avocado or mayonnaise), and one California roll (no avocado or mayonnaise).

Meal Four: Meal replacement drink.

Meal Five: Try one of the many pizza recipes found in the recipe chapter.

Your Day Seventeen Workout

1. Are you ready to pump up again? Today, you're going to do fourteen Sixty-Second Workouts. Make sure to include stretches.

2. For extra credit, try a different light cardio activity.

Evening Pep Talk

You can't eliminate all the negative people in your life who might envy what you're doing, but the fact is that most people, deep down, have great admiration for those who hold fast to this program. So tonight, congratulate yourself. Take some pride in what you're doing. And vow to yourself that, starting tomorrow, you won't feel the slightest embarrassment in social situations when you tell others about what the Slimdown for Life is doing for you. Tell them about the way you have fit proper eating and fitness into your lifestyle. Share the stories of your own success. I think you'll be astounded at the crowd that gathers around you.

As a matter of fact, I want you to go so far as to make sure others know *how important you are to yourself*! I'm not telling you to be arrogant and self-absorbed. But how you act determines how others react to you. To be important to others, you must think you're important. To gain the respect of others, you must first act as if you deserve respect. It's that simple: The more respect you have for yourself, the more respect others will have for you.

Slimdown Tip: Making "Better Bad Choices"

My friend, the well-known Houston nutritionist Keith Klein, has invented a great phrase to describe another way to cheat. He calls it making "Better Bad Choices." These are foods that won't get you leaner, but certainly will prevent you from getting too much fatter. They are the foods you look for when you're at a sporting event or movie theater—someplace where you're stuck with a very fixed menu, almost all of it high in fat. There are going to be times when you reach certain emotional states—a terrible day at the office, for example, or for women it may be PMS—and you will come home and see food as a sort of salve. You know these kinds of days: You want a big helping of good old fattening "comfort food." This is when you need to have the right kinds of Better Bad Choices in your kitchen—sugar-free Popsicles instead of ice cream bars, dried fruit instead of candy, fat-free brownies instead of cookies, and baked potato chips instead of fried potato chips. If you're going to pig out on potato chips, then at least pig out on the ones with the fewest calories. Or if you need a big dessert, look at items such as the Key Lime Pie and the Banana Pudding in the recipe chapter. You literally will have trouble telling that they are low fat.

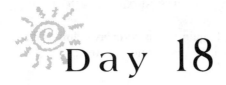

Day 18

Fighting Your First Backslide

Today is one of the most important days of the Slimdown for Life because it's going to be your security blanket. We're going to talk about the moment that could come in the future when you stop doing the program. For whatever reason, you quit following the Slimdown— and you've got to convince yourself to get started again.

"No, Larry, it will never happen to me," you might be saying. "I'm committed to the Slimdown." And I know you are. But there is a chance some of you will backslide at some point in the future. That's why this day is so important—so you'll know what to do. Your first backslide on this program is going to be one of your biggest challenges. If you handle your first slip successfully, you're much more likely to be able to recover from future slips.

Here's how a typical backslide works. If you go through a period in your life where things are hectic, you might decide to go off the program for a day. Then you might put it off a second day, which makes its easier to put it off a third day, as you say to yourself, "Well, let me get the rest of my life in order—let me get all my projects done—and then I'll really get back on the program." What's happening is that the backslide is turning into an avalanche. Suddenly, the whole idea of getting started again seems so overwhelming that you put off the program even another week.

How to Get Back Up

Have you never noticed that one of the toughest things to do in life is get out of a warm bed into a cold room? The longer you lie there and think how unpleasant it will be to get up, the more difficult it becomes. But there's no way around it. You have to throw off the covers and put your feet on the floor. And once you do it—once you take the first small step out of bed—you realize that it was not that difficult to get out of bed.

It's the same thing with a backslide. The longer you wait, the harder it is to get started again. So don't wait even one extra minute to begin your recovery. Put aside any disappointment, frustration, or anger you are feeling with yourself, because that only postpones the effort you must make.

And always, always, start back in small ways. Take small steps just as you did at the very start of the program. Don't demand perfection of yourself right after a setback. Don't set unrealistic goals for yourself to try to "catch up." Far too many people set themselves up for greater failure after a relapse by imposing strict rules and guidelines that cannot be followed for life. This program is a lifelong journey, not an overnight trip. Like any road you travel down, there will be bumps, red lights, yellow lights, detours, and unexpected stops.

I would suggest you review what you learned in the first week of this program. Go back and look at the first week of the program and then set up an easy day of eating and exercising for yourself. Take a look at your

Personal Mission Statement again. You also might take out a sheet of paper, mark a vertical line down the middle, and in the left-hand column, list all the benefits of sticking to the Slimdown for Life. Write down anything that comes to your mind. ("I've already lost fifteen pounds. I have more energy," etc.) On the right side of the page, write down all the consequences you know will come if you continue to backslide. ("I'll be out of shape. My belly will come back," etc.) You might also want to spread around some "motivation." Put a Post-it Note on your bathroom mirror with a sentence on it about achieving your dreams. Stick a note to the refrigerator door about the wonderful things that a properly balanced meal will do for your body.

Your Day Eighteen
Eating Guide

Meal One: Four scrambled egg whites and French toast.

Meal Two: Turkey sandwich.

Meal Three: Eat out at an Italian restaurant. Try grilled chicken breast (ask that it be cooked with no oil but be sure to have a few wedges of lemon on the side), one small side dish of pasta (keep it to a few ounces) with marinara sauce, and a Caesar salad with dressing on the side.

Meal Four: Chicken breast, potato, and fibrous veggie.

Meal Five: Baked fish, saffron rice, and salad with fat-free dressing.

Your Day Eighteen Workout

1. Once again, complete fourteen Sixty-Second Workouts.
2. A thirty-minute walk.

Evening Pep Talk

Now here's the most important thing to do when you backslide. Make sure you do at least *one* thing before the day is over to help you get back on the program. Don't make the mistake of telling yourself at the start of the day that you're going to do something and then not keep your word. As odd as this sounds, it's very important early on in this program to establish trust with yourself. Each time you break a promise to yourself, you chip away at the supply of your own trust until you eventually get to the point where you are plagued by self-doubt.

Let's say that you get up in the morning with the goal of doing some exercising, but as the day goes on, you say, "I'm too tired. I'll work out later." When "later" comes, you still don't do anything, but this time you say, "I'll do it the first thing tomorrow morning." When tomorrow morning comes, you think, "I have too much to do. I'll wait until this weekend." And so on. After a few times of doing this, you'll develop such a negative mind-set that you might stop believing you can accomplish whatever it is you want. Then you're in danger of letting your backslide turn into a total collapse.

So when the backslide comes, make a small promise to yourself about how you'll recover for that day and then keep your promise, whether it means taking a short walk or eating one good meal. If you have to, do one Sixty-Second Workout tonight before you go to bed. It's a way of letting your subconscious know that you're still serious about getting lean and staying lean. If you wish, zero in on one aspect of the program that you really want to focus on that day, and then after you have kept your promise, congratulate yourself for having done what you said you would do. When getting back on the program after a backslide, it is better to make fewer commitments and keep the ones that you make rather than making too many and breaking them. Let me tell you, after all the work you did last week on thinking and acting in a positive manner, you do not want get back in the position of being overcome by negative thoughts.

Slimdown Tip: Using Salt

I don't worry all that much about salt. Why? The table salt that you add to food is not the culprit when it comes to high sodium in this country. It's the fast food and processed food and greasy food that Americans eat. It you eat according to the guidelines of this program, you will not be using highly salty foods. (If you are pregnant, you need to watch your salt intake, and if you have high blood pressure, you should, of course, cut back on salt.) I don't suggest you dump a lot of salt on your food, but a light sprinkling is okay. Salt is a great flavor enhancer.

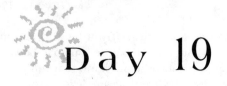

Day 19

Building Back a Positive Attitude

If you backslide on the Slimdown for Life, I want you to be as understanding with yourself as you would be with a beloved child. Don't for one minute think about how "bad" you are if you slip off the program. The more you let that negative voice into your life, the more it will urge you into even more destructive behavior. Listening to that voice often can make you your own worst enemy.

A weak period is exactly the time when you cannot—I repeat, cannot—allow negative thoughts about failure to enter your brain. What I want you to do is . . . smile! That's right. This is not a program designed to create demeaning self-reprimands. This is a program to make you feel good about your life. So always keep your sense of humor. You make a mistake? Not to worry. You've got tomorrow to get better.

When I go through low periods and lack my usual enthusiasm, I do my best to be around very positive and supportive people. I would recommend you do the same thing. They can be the best way for you to stay centered on your goals.

Positive attitudes are contagious. When looking toward the future, negative people often foresee gloom and doom. But positive people are different. They don't wear rose-colored glasses, but they never lose sight or hope. Associating with positive people makes you think more positively. With them, the future always holds hope, and it's that very hope that leads to change. The more positive friendships you cultivate, the better off you'll be maintaining your own positive attitude, regardless what happens in your life.

Using Visualizations

Remember how we talked about visualizations? Visualizations of who you want to be are perfect techniques for dealing with social pressure. During weak periods, I work harder than ever at visualizing myself at my absolute best. It is a technique used all the time by professional athletes who get into slumps. A baseball player who is in a hitting slump, for example, envisions himself taking his stance in the batter's box, watching the pitcher wind up, following the ball toward home plate, swinging at the ball, connecting, and watching it go over the fence for a home run. He visualizes this scene over and over and over. Researchers call this "cognitive restructuring," and it really works. Golfers imagine hitting the perfect golf shot to help them improve their swing, and basketball players imagine making fifty free throws in a row, using perfect form. You, too, can use visualizations to imagine yourself following the program perfectly. By running a kind of home movie about yourself in your brain, then you will develop renewed confidence. You can visualize yourself eating a perfectly balanced meal. You can visualize yourself doing twenty

Sixty-Second Workouts. You can visualize yourself at the perfect weight.

Don't be skeptical. Researchers know these visualizations work. They work because they motivate you to turn them into a reality. They help bring back your self-esteem. They make you realize, once again, that you can be in control. All you have to do is relax and let the positive part of your mind work for you. Your mind is much stronger than you can ever imagine.

Here's a sample visualization: Imagine looking at your body in the mirror and smiling because you are a lean, thin, vibrant person. Imagine yourself in the kind of form-fitting clothes you've always wanted to wear. Imagine yourself possessing the elegant muscle tone that you've always wanted. Imagine the inside of your body operating as a beautiful clean engine, running on the purest of fuel.

Do you see? When you create such visualizations in your head, you're not just daydreaming. You're really doing something to make your dreams come true.

Your Day Nineteen Eating Guide

Meal One: Cereal with skim milk, sprinkled with fruit.

Meal Two: Meal replacement drink.

Meal Three: Eat out at a Mexican restaurant. Try grilled chicken fajitas (ask that they be cooked with no oil), corn tortillas (not flour), lettuce, onion, tomatoes, and rice.

Meal Four: A half cup of yogurt mixed with a half cup of oats and a piece of fruit.

Meal Five: Grilled chicken, potato or rice, and salad with fat-free dressing.

Your Day Nineteen Workout

1. Now we're up to fifteen Sixty-Second Workouts. This is your last hard workout day, and we're ratcheting up the number of workouts just to give your muscles an extra push.

2. Walk thirty to sixty minutes.

Evening Pep Talk

Do you remember how I told you at the start of the book that this is a program about progress, not perfection? It's true. I'm never expecting you to get through this program perfectly. If you do this program at only 50 percent, you'll still make progress.

What I care most deeply about is that you don't get discouraged. You can have some kind of backslide every single day, but as long as you're doing the program in some fashion—any kind of fashion—you're doing a lot better for yourself than you were before you started this program. That's what matters to me.

So stay positive. Be proud of yourself. Smile. As time goes on, there might be more relapses, but the great news is that there will always be even more progress—*as long as you keep trying.* That's all it takes.

Slimdown Tip: Smoking and Weight Loss

Many of you are smokers, and you know that in the past when you've quit smoking, you've had a tendency to gain lots of weight. I expect some of you are wondering if you should be especially afraid of doing the Slimdown program because of all the food you are eating. The answer: absolutely not. The reason smokers gain weight is not because they have quit smoking. It's because they have begun eating *more* of the same fatty, processed foods they've always eaten. If a smoker quits smoking and goes on this type of eating program, he or she will lose fat and increase in lean muscle tissue. The simple solution to losing weight after having smoked is to follow this program—nothing more, nothing less.

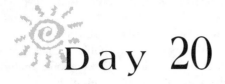

Day 20

A Final Review of What You've Learned

Today, as we come to the close of these three weeks, I want you to look back through the all the previous pages and review what you have learned. In all honesty, you have been given an amazing amount of information. I don't expect you to remember all of it, of course—just as long as you remember the program's basic cornerstones that will last you a lifetime.

1. Eat five meals a day, one every three to four hours.
2. If at all possible, each meal should contain a serving of lean protein and a serving of starchy carbs, with a fibrous vegetable thrown in whenever you wish.
3. The lean protein should be about the size of your hand, the starchy carb should be about the size of your fist, and the fibrous vegetable should fit into a cereal bowl.
4. Gradually reduce as much dietary fat out of your food as possible. Recognize that you will be getting enough fat in the healthful foods that you will be eating on this program. The more fat you reduce, the quicker your body loses body fat.
5. Maintain a walking program, three to four times a week, in which each walk lasts thirty to sixty minutes.
6. To tone your muscle tissue, which is where the

most calories and fat can be burned, do up to twelve Sixty-Second Workouts every day, half of which should work your upper body, half your lower body. Include stretches to give your muscle tissue elasticity.

That's all there is to it. That's all you need to remember. The Slimdown for Life is simple, reliable, and effective. By regulating your meals every three hours, you are preventing your body's digestive system from being overly swamped with food, thus preventing the excess calories from flooding your fat cells. By eating lean proteins, starchy carbs, and fibrous vegetables, you are feeding your body only the most healthful foods, which will bypass the fat cells if taken in the proper amounts. And by cutting back on dietary fat, you are cutting back on the unhealthful foods, which truly make you fat. Finally, your walking program will burn the fat in your body, and your Sixty-Second Workouts will build the muscle so that you can burn even more calories.

Your Day Twenty Eating Guide

Meal One: Egg muffin and one cup of oatmeal.

Meal Two: Chicken breast and rice.

Meal Three: Eat at an Asian restaurant. Try a shrimp spring roll (not fried), grilled lemon grass chicken, and rice noodles, or a similar combination.

Meal Four: Egg white omelette, and one cup of creamed rice cereal.

Meal Five: Pasta with Ham and Peas from the recipe chapter.

Your Day Twenty Workout

1. Complete a total of twelve Sixty-Second Workouts.
2. Walk for forty-five to sixty minutes.

Evening Pep Talk

As you go to bed tonight, I want you to say three words out loud—moderation, balance, and steadiness. Yeah, yeah, I know, they are very boring words for a pep talk. But as you know, they have been the keys to your success. You cannot follow an eating and fitness program for the rest of your life that forces you to act in an extreme manner. I said it at the start of the book, and I'll say it again here: Any program that you can't do for the rest of your life is not worth doing for a single day. If you want to be successful, you must commit yourself to taking small steps—steps that require moderation, balance, and steadiness. It's because of these words that you will be able to transform your body, to shed your old identity and step forth boldly into the future. You might not see it yet, but these small steps are growing larger and larger and the results becoming more tangible. Just as a downhill skier starts off slowly at the top of the hill but quickly becomes unstoppable as he progresses down the slope, so, too, are you building momentum to reach your ultimate goal of a lean, healthy body.

Slimdown Tip:
Getting Tighter Abs

Many of you are getting great results on the program, but you're wondering if there is something extra you can do to get a tighter stomach. You are doing all the stomach crunches described in the exercise chapter, but you just can't seem to get rid of the fat around your midsection. I'm sorry to tell you this, but doing sit-ups and stomach crunches or any other abdominal exercise is a pure waste of time when it comes to removing the extra fat around your middle. That doesn't mean abdominal work isn't good for you. It tightens your muscles there so you do look fitter. But the only way to lose the inner tube around your waist is through the Slimdown's eating program, and the eating program alone. An increase in your cardio activity can help slightly, but the true secret is to cheat less and reduce the foods you're not supposed to eat. All in all, there is no exercise substitute for the eating program.

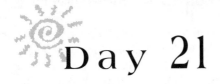

Day 21

Your Day of Victory

What can I say? Right now, I'm almost speechless. You have turned little steps into great strides because of your simple but noble decision to make a better life for yourself. Opening the door and stepping out of your past required a commitment that most people don't have. You made the decision to fly adventurously into the unknown.

There is really nothing more I can tell you. It is so moving for me to see how much you have accomplished on this program. You know exactly what to do to make your body leaner and stronger. You've learned all the keys to being fit and to keeping bad food out of your life without feeling the slightest bit deprived. In so many ways, you have honored yourself. As time goes on, I want you to remember that. You have worked so hard at learning to believe in yourself. With your newfound control and discipline, you are already exhibiting a kind of enthusiasm and passion that others haven't seen in you before.

How Far This Program Can Take You

I get letters from young mothers, business executives, grandparents, students. All of them have stories to tell about the way the program has helped give them the strength and confidence to be able to create a much better life for themselves. I remember once talking to a land surveyor named Willie. When I met him, he weighed 435 pounds. One day he blacked out at his job site, was sent to the hospital, and was told by his doctor, "Willie, you can either lose weight, or you can die." Willie heard about the Slimdown for Life, started following the program, and ended up losing 135 pounds in less than eight months. (You can see his testimony in my infomercial.) A year later, he had lost another 90 pounds, discovered to his astonishment that there was a woman who loved him, and married her.

I said, "Willie, has there been any downside to the program?"

He said, "Larry, the program has slowed down my work output."

"What do you mean?" I asked, a little baffled.

"I have trouble getting work done because so many people come up to me asking if I will tell them about this program I found to help me lose weight."

There was Sandy Friesenhahn, a North Dallas housewife who had been chubby almost her entire life. She thought she had no time for herself—she was working two jobs *and* taking care of kids. But then her wake-up call came. She told me she had to do something—anything—to feel confident about herself. She was tired of feeling embarrassed in public about the way she looked. She didn't have time to go a gym, she later told me, and she didn't have time to whip up perfect low-fat meals. But she took my program, learned how to get in her five daily meals simply and quickly, learned to get in her workouts, and lost so much weight and body fat that many people who saw her in a swimsuit told her she should enter a beauty pageant. Sandy did . . . and became the Mrs. Texas Runner-Up.

Let me tell you one final story about the power of this program. I will never forget how I was doing one of my live weekly radio broadcasts at a shopping mall, and a man walked up who looked vaguely familiar. I kept staring at him. Then it hit me. It was the most feared coach from my high school. When I attended high school, Coach truly made my life miserable. He had a crewcut, a very bulky physical presence, and a fiercely intimidating and somewhat redneck manner. At the time, I was a boy who had just moved from New York and I was completely out of place in Dallas. I wore a black T-shirt over my soft, flabby body, and I wore an earring as a fashion statement. I don't have to tell you that the coach found me completely irritating from the moment he laid eyes on me. He instructed the high school football team that if they were seen talking to me or befriending me, they would do extra laps at practice.

Part of the joy of leaving high school, I thought, was getting away from that coach. And then, after years and years, there he was standing in front of me. Although I was by then considered a national fitness expert, I reverted right back to my adolescent state. "Oh, my God," I thought, "what is he going to do?"

Coach took the microphone, which was available for the audience, and he asked, "Do you remember who I am?"

"Yes, sir," I said, my voice shaking.

"Well," he said, "I drove down here to tell your listeners something. I came here to say that I once made your life miserable, and I'm now here to ask your forgiveness. I was recently diagnosed with cancer, and my doctor said, 'You need to follow this Larry North program, because he has the right idea on getting fit and eating right.'"

The coach paused. "And I'm here to tell your listeners, this program saved my life. I have gotten healthier than I have ever been before. I have a newfound sense of energy. And I feel like I'm beating the cancer. Larry, I believe my success is because of this program."

Then he gave me a smile, turned on his heels, and slowly walked away. I never saw or heard from him again.

I know that's a dramatic story. Your own story of success, of course, is probably nothing like that. I know for many of you, the success will be the great relief that comes when you realize you have found a way to get lean permanently without having to torture yourself. I can't tell you the number of times people have come up to me on the street and said, "Larry, I'm on Day Sixteen." Or "Larry, I just finished your twenty-one days." Or "Larry, I've been on the program for a year and I'm going stronger than ever before."

So stay with it. Get up every morning with a fierce desire to stoke the furnace inside your body, to feed that furnace with the best fuel, and to take the time for more workouts to make that furnace burn off any excess fat hanging around. You, too, will soon realize this exhilaration does not end. The more success you see, the more success you will want. You will *want* to find extra ways to get lean. You will *want* to do the one little thing at each meal to cut out some excess fat calories. You will *want* to spend ten extra minutes walking. Indeed, you will be so full of energy—which is something that I know you never got on a standard "diet"—that you will set even more stringent goals for yourself so that you can become leaner and healthier every day.

Your Day Twenty-one Eating Guide

Meal One: Four to six scrambled egg whites and one cup of baked hash browns.

Meal Two: Grilled chicken sandwich.

Meal Three: Grilled flounder, potato, and a vegetable.

Meal Four: Meal replacement drink.

Meal Five: To celebrate the end of the three weeks, treat yourself to a great steak dinner. Order a filet mignon, from one to six ounces, one baked potato with everything on the side, a dinner salad with fat-free dressing on the side, and sliced beefsteak tomatoes.

Your Day Twenty-one Workout

You'll love this. After all the work you've done this week, treat yourself to a day of rest. In fact, give yourself a reward. See today's Slimdown Tip.

Evening Pep Talk

Remember that bottle of champagne I told you to buy when we were just starting this book? It's time to open it. As we conclude, I want you to know how, from the very bottom of my heart, I am honored to have had this opportunity to work with you.

I think one of the reasons the world is so full of frustrated people is that they know they have great potential, but tragically, they have never stuck to their vision of what they could become. It is not that they don't want to change, but they don't want to commit to change. They look at people like you and think that you must be "very lucky" to have found such a niche. They are probably asking themselves, "How did you get so lucky?"

Hey, as you know, luck had nothing to do with it. You simply made a decision to change—and then you stayed committed to change. It's that commitment to continue to change that makes you so special!

I know this is the end of the book, but it is really just the beginning. Have you ever heard the saying, "Today is the first day of the rest of your life"? That's exactly where you are. In so many ways, your journey is just beginning. All you have to do is keep believing in yourself and keep believing in this program, and the journey will take you places that you cannot imagine and lead you to horizons you never knew existed.

I wish you Godspeed and bon voyage.

Slimdown Tip: Give Yourself a Workout Reward

Because you've been pushing yourself harder this week physically than you have in a long time, it's time to treat your body with a little TLC. Tender loving care. You can take a long luxuriating bath or pamper yourself at a hair salon, but I'd like to suggest something that makes you feel better than ever about your body. Have a professional masseur give you a soothing, uplifting massage.

A professional massage costs money, but it's amazing how it will connect you to your body. During a massage, the points of tension and stress in your body seemingly disappear. If you're in deep stress, it can help you relax. It also helps prevent injury by working out some of the pain in your body. It is a remarkably healthy endeavor. And, you feel pampered with the soothing strokes of the masseur. For overweight people especially, the experience of being touched and pampered can be so nourishing. After a massage, you will really love your body and be more attuned to taking care of it.

Part Three

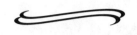

Staying the Course

You don't just finish this program. You only get better at it.

Most Frequently Asked Questions

I'm following your program, but I'm gaining weight—and I'm worried I'm eating too much food. What is happening to me?

I hear this question all the time, and I have one question in response. Are you really following the program, or are you faking it? When people tell me they are gaining weight on the program, I make them go through a detailed description of their meals. It invariably becomes clear they are not eating right. They are skipping meals regularly or eating only a banana or muffin for breakfast or eating huge dinners that saturate their fat cells. Many of you tend to forget that you can eat too much good food and still get fat. You have to eat the correct portion sizes. So make sure your portion sizes are exactly right, and make sure you are not snacking on high-fat foods in between meals.

Well, my problem is not that I'm gaining weight. It's that I'm not dropping weight as fast as I thought I should be. So what should I do?

Before you do a thing, ask yourself a few questions: Is your energy increasing? Do you have more endurance? Are you getting stronger? Do you feel good about the foods that you are eating? And finally, do you feel you are losing inches? The last question is the key. In this program, we always lose in inches, not pounds. We lose body fat, not just body weight. The lean muscle tissue you're adding to your body weighs more than your body fat, so it might not look like you've lost great amounts of weight. But you will look amazingly better. Even then, if you stick with the program, making sure you keep your meals regulated and your portions at their right size, you'll ultimately lose all the weight that you want.

I'd like to be on your program, but it seems like it's way too expensive to eat this much food.

Actually, this program is the most economical program you'll ever go on in your life. There are no packaged foods or expensive supplements you need to order the way you do on commercial diets. And the staples of this program are very cheap. My wife and I do a lot of our shopping at warehouse supermarkets, and we can buy a twenty-five-pound bag of rice for five dollars, a sack of twenty potatoes for less than twenty cents a potato, a package of ten boned and skinned chicken breasts for a dollar a breast, and fresh, frozen, and canned vegetables for as little as fifteen cents a serving. Many of my meals throughout the day cost less than two dollars per meal. Where else can you get a complete meal so inexpensively?

How can a vegetarian do this program?

The rules stay the same. You want to try to eat five balanced meals a day of lean proteins and starchy carbs. If you are the type of vegetarian who can incorporate egg whites, fish, and protein powders into your diet, then you'll do just fine. If you are a classic "vegan" who eats no animal products at all, you can combine certain foods to give yourself protein, such as rice and beans, but it is going to be more difficult for you. My recommendation is to spread your meals out through the day and get in what combinations of protein you can.

How can a diabetic do this program?

If you are a diabetic, you should, of course, check first and foremost with your physician about this program. However, when it comes to regulating your blood sugar levels, you will never find a program better suited for diabetics. Think about what you're being told to do: Eat every three hours. Eat high-quality foods that combine protein and carbs, and reduce sugars, fats, and processed foods.

Can a pregnant woman do this program?

Again, check first with your doctor. But I think he or she would tell you that there is no better time in your life to get healthy and fit than when you become pregnant. With a few modifications and dietary supplements the eating program is perfect for you and your baby.

I've been on the program for a few months, and I've lost over thirty pounds. I feel that I look better, but now I want to move forward. How do I go on to the next level and get that lean, toned body that you see on so many movie stars and athletes?

Quite often, even when we've made tremendous progress, we tend to still be very subjective with our own bodies—and we want to figure out ways to get better. If your goal is now to get a much harder body, then it's time to make a move into a gym or health club. I'll be very honest: I think you ought to hire an experienced personal trainer who can lead you into a more advanced fitness program that will keep you from working out too hard or getting an injury.

8

The Seven-Day Sizedown

Many times I have had people say to me that they have a wedding to go to within a week, or they've just been invited on a weekend beach trip, or a class reunion is coming up that they want to look their best for. They give me this desperate look and ask what they can do to lose as much weight as possible in seven days.

Well, of course, they could fast—which would be unhealthy and would backfire on them in a couple of days when they go on a massive eating binge. But I have developed a very extreme, hard-core version of the Slimdown for Life, which I call the Seven-Day Sizedown. It might come in handy for you someday, but please, please, don't misconstrue this as the best way to work your normal program. It is a quick fix. It is practically impossible to do longer than seven days. It's too strict for me to do for very long.

But if you want to go to the wall every now and then and try to strip off as much fat as you can as quickly as possible, I will show you what to do.

Let me warn you at the start. Do not use this program for more than seven days and be sure to take vitamin and mineral supplements. There is absolutely no cheating on the Seven-Day Sizedown. If you make any mistake or try to slip in any bad foods, you're not going to get the results. You might as well stay on the normal program. You have to eat exactly the foods I tell you to eat. You have to do as much exercise as I tell you to do. And you must cut all fat, all oil, all sugar, and even diet sodas. If at all possible, make your beverages nothing but water.

Are you still interested? Okay, here we go:

Seven-Day Sizedown Menu

You will eat the same set of meals every day for the next seven days. No substitions or additions allowed. Women will change their Meal Five slightly, and there is one extra meal at the end of the day for men only.

Meal One: Six hard-boiled egg whites and one cup of cream of rice cereal.

Meal Two: One grilled chicken breast with one cup of steamed vegetable and one cup of brown rice.

Meal Three: Same as Meal Two.

Meal Four: Six hard-boiled egg whites and one cup of cream of rice cereal.

Meal Five: Baked or broiled white meat fish with a plain baked potato and a veggie. (For women, cut the potato and replace with a cup of a second fibrous vegetable.)

Meal Six: For men only. A meal later in the night consisting of a protein and a fibrous veggie. No starchy carb.

It's okay to season your food with dry spices except salt and sugar.

Snacking and Eating Out

If you must snack, eat only crunchy vegetables and a piece of fruit or two each day. But under no circumstances do you miss a meal. If you know you're not going to be able to be home for a meal, then you *must* bring a perfectly balanced meal with you.

One more no-no. Do not eat at any restaurant. There's too great of a chance that they'll slip some fat into your food. If you're having an emergency and must get your meal in, then go to a Chinese restaurant, order steamed rice, steamed white meat skinless chicken, and a steamed vegetable. Do not allow any oil to be used on your food.

Seven-Day Sizedown Workouts

1. On the first, third, fifth, and seventh days—in other words, every other day—you will do fifteen Sixty-Second Workouts.

2. You will walk every single day, between forty-five and sixty minutes.

Plain and simple, this is a raw, no-nonsense week of perfect eating. Still, if you need to lose a lot of pounds in a hurry, this is what to do. It remains a far superior option than a food-depriving diet.

CHAPTER

9

Slimdown Recipes

Throughout the book, I wanted to give you a combination of fast, easy-to-cook dishes (which you've found spread throughout your Eating Guides each day). Here, you will find some easy dishes and other dishes that are really special, wondrously tasty, and incredibly devoid of fat.

Breakfast Dishes

French Toast

YIELD: **4** SERVINGS

Ingredients:

3 Egg Beaters®
½ cup skim milk
3 tablespoons sugar
½ teaspoon cinnamon or nutmeg

8 slices of bread
Lemon
Powdered sugar

Cooking Instructions:

Preheat a nonstick skillet or griddle to medium heat. Beat the Egg Beaters® and milk together with the sugar and cinnamon. Dip bread into egg mixture. Place bread on hot skillet and cook until lightly browned. Flip and continue cooking until brown. Sprinkle with powdered sugar and squeeze of lemon.

Egg Muffins

YIELD: **4** SERVINGS

Ingredients:

8 egg whites
1 teaspoon butter substitute such as Butter Buds®
Salt, pepper, onion powder, and garlic powder
Sautéed mushrooms, onions, and green peppers (optional)

4 English muffins, each one split in half
4 slices fat-free American cheese
4 slices lean Canadian bacon or smoked turkey

Cooking Instructions:

Combine the egg whites with the seasonings. Beat to mix well. Remove both top and bottom lids from an empty tuna can and rinse well. Heat a nonstick skillet or one sprayed with nonstick spray until hot over medium heat. Place the tuna can in it and carefully pour in the egg mixture. Reduce the heat to low and cover. Cook 5 to 7 minutes, or until done. Remove and run a knife around the edge to loosen the egg patty. Toast the English muffin, if desired, and place the ham, egg, and cheese on top. Store in zipper bags in refrigerator. To reheat the refrigerated muffins, microwave 20 to 30 seconds on high.

Power Muffins

YIELD: 12 SERVINGS

Ingredients:

2 cups rolled oats
10 egg whites
2 apples, peeled and chopped
1 teaspoon cinnamon
½ teaspoon vanilla

3 packages Sweet 'n' Low (not Equal®) or 3 teaspoons honey
1 teaspoon grated orange or lemon rind
½ cup raisins

Cooking Instructions:

Preheat oven to 375 degrees. Combine all ingredients and beat with an electric mixer for two minutes. Pour into nonstick muffin pans. Bake in preheated oven for 15 to 20 minutes. Store in zipper bags in refrigerator. To reheat the refrigerated muffins, microwave 20 to 30 seconds on high.

Cheese Grits

YIELD: 4 SERVINGS

Ingredients:

2 cups water
½ cup quick cooking grits
Pinch of salt
1 tablespoon minced dried
 onion

4 ounces fat-free cheddar
 slices torn into pieces
Dash of garlic powder
2 drops hot pepper sauce

Cooking Instructions:

Bring water to a boil. Add grits, salt, and dried minced onion. Stir to mix well, and cook 5 minutes. Stir in torn-up cheese slices, garlic, and hot pepper sauce. Remove from heat and serve.

Salads

Fiesta Bean and Corn Salad

YIELD: **1 2** SERVINGS

Ingredients:

1 medium onion, chopped
2 tomatoes, chopped
1 pound frozen corn,
   defrosted
1 jalapeño, chopped
1 15-ounce can black or
   pinto beans, drained
   and rinsed

3–4 tablespoons fresh
   squeezed lime juice
1 tablespoon red wine
   vinegar
½ teaspoon pepper
1 teaspoon salt
⅓ cup fresh cilantro,
   chopped

Preparation:

Combine all the ingredients in a bowl. Mix well. Cover and refrigerate for 30 minutes to let the flavors develop. Serve with baked corn tortilla chips.

Taco Salad

YIELD: **3 – 4** SERVINGS

Ingredients:

1 pound 90–95% lean
   ground beef or pure
   ground turkey breast
1 package taco seasoning
   mix

Water, to achieve desired
   consistency

Cooking Instructions:

In a large skillet, brown the ground meat. When it is almost completely cooked, run the hot water in your sink. Place the completely cooked meat into a colander and rinse under the running hot water for a couple of minutes. Rinse out your skillet also. Reheat your skillet on medium high; return the meat to the skillet along with the taco seasoning. Stir together with about ½ cup water and simmer about 5 minutes.

To make the Taco Salad itself, put a layer of corn chips in a bowl. Sprinkle on about a quarter of the meat. Add ½ head of chopped iceberg lettuce, 2 chopped tomatoes, ½ pound shredded fat-free cheddar cheese, ½ chopped onion, and hot sauce. Dab on a couple tablespoons of fat-free sour cream and sprinkle on a teaspoon of chopped cilantro.

Broccoli-Cauliflower Salad

YIELD: 4 – 6 SERVINGS

Ingredients:

1 head cauliflower	*1 medium red onion*
1 bunch broccoli	*1 small jar pimentos*

To make the dressing, combine the following:

1 cup fat-free mayonnaise *or salad dressing*	*¼ cup vinegar*
1–2 tablespoons sugar	*1 tablespoon dry mustard*
	Salt and pepper to taste

Preparation:

Combine the dressing ingredients and set aside. Clean the cauliflower and broccoli and cut into florets. Chop the onion. In a large bowl, combine the vegetables with the pimentos and toss with the dressing. Marinate overnight for best flavor.

Mushroom and Hearts Salad

YIELD: 4 – 6 SERVINGS

Ingredients:

1 pound sliced mushrooms
1 can artichoke hearts
  (smallest hearts
  possible—highest
  number of hearts per
  can)

1 can or jar hearts of palm
1 clove garlic, minced
Juice of 1½ lemons
½ teaspoon each salt and
  pepper

Preparation:

Rinse the mushrooms. Slice the artichokes into quarters or bite-sized pieces. Slice the hearts of palm into quarter rounds. Combine the mushrooms, artichokes, hearts of palm, and garlic in a bowl. Pour lemon juice over all and sprinkle with salt and pepper. Toss to mix well. Refrigerate for an hour to marinate before serving.

Rice Salad

YIELD: 4 SERVINGS

Ingredients:

*8 ounces fresh mushrooms,
    sliced*
¼ cup chicken broth
1 cup frozen corn
2 cups cooked rice, cold
*4 boneless, skinless chicken
    breasts, cooked and
    diced*
1 green bell pepper, diced
1 medium onion, diced

*1 can Le Sueur peas,
    drained*
1 small jar diced pimentos
1 cup fat-free mayonnaise
*½ cup fat-free vinaigrette
    (recipe below)*
½ teaspoon garlic powder
½ teaspoon onion powder
Salt and pepper, to taste
2 ripe tomatoes, diced

Preparation:

Sauté mushrooms in chicken broth until soft and slightly brown around the edges. Remove from heat and place in a large bowl. Warm corn in the same pan. Drain and combine with mushrooms. Add rice, chicken, green pepper, onion, peas, pimento, mayonnaise, and vinaigrette. Put in seasonings and adjust to taste. Cover with plastic wrap and refrigerate overnight for best flavor. Before serving, add tomatoes. Toss to mix well.

To make the fat-free vinaigrette:

Mix ¼–⅓ cup red wine vinegar, 1 teaspoon Italian herb seasoning (crushed), ¼ cup skim milk, 1–2 teaspoons Dijon mustard, and salt, pepper, garlic, and onion powder to taste.

Appetizers
and Snacks

Seven-Layer Dip

YIELD: 10 – 12 SERVINGS

Ingredients:

1 15-ounce can fat-free
  refried beans
1 recipe asparagus
  guacamole (see
  following recipe)
1 package taco seasoning
  (optional)
1 cup fat-free sour cream

1 cup grated fat-free cheddar
  cheese
1 large tomato, diced
1 bunch green onions,
  chopped, green part
  only
1 jalapeño pepper, sliced or
  chopped

Preparation:

Evenly spread beans in the bottom of an 8x8-inch glass
baking dish. Spread a layer of asparagus guacamole on
top of the beans. Mix the taco seasoning with the sour
cream and spread on top of the guacamole. Sprinkle
the cheese on top. Sprinkle diced tomatoes, then the
green onions and the jalapeño. Serve with fat-free tortilla chips.

Asparagus Guacamole

YIELD: 4 – 6 SERVINGS

Ingredients:

1 14-ounce can asparagus, drained

1 cup tomato, diced and seeded (about 1 large tomato)

⅓ cup onion, diced

2 tablespoons fat-free mayonnaise or Miracle Whip®

2 tablespoons cilantro, minced

1 tablespoon lime juice, freshly squeezed

6 drops red pepper sauce

1 clove garlic, minced

¼ cup picante sauce, drained of excess liquid

Preparation:

Process the asparagus until smooth. Combine with all other ingredients, cover, and refrigerate at least 1 hour. Serve with baked corn tortilla chips.

Try it with fat-free sour cream instead of mayonnaise. Canned asparagus is the key; fresh or frozen just doesn't have the right texture (mush).

Artichoke Spread

YIELD: 10 – 12 SERVINGS

Ingredients:

18 ounces artichoke hearts, canned in water

½ teaspoon lemon zest, finely grated

½ teaspoon garlic powder

½ teaspoon Italian herb seasonings

½ cup mild, soft, low-fat goat cheese

½ cup fat-free plain yogurt

2 tablespoons Italian parsley (flat leaf), finely chopped

1½ teaspoons pepper, coarsely ground

Several drops Tabasco® Sauce

Preparation:

Drain and coarsely chop artichokes and toss with lemon zest, garlic powder, and Italian seasonings. Process goat cheese and yogurt together in a blender. Season, then fold everything together, cover, and refrigerate for 2 hours.

Deviled Eggs

YIELD: 10 SERVINGS

Ingredients:

1 can white beans, rinsed
    and drained
4 tablespoons minced onion
1 tablespoon mustard
½ cup fat-free mayonnaise
Paprika

Several drops Tabasco®
    Sauce
2 tablespoons sweet relish
Salt and pepper, to taste
10 hard-boiled eggs, sliced
    in half lengthwise
Curry powder

Preparation:

Purée the beans in a food processor. Add the onion, mustard, mayonnaise, paprika, and Tabasco®. Process until well mixed. Stir in the relish, and add salt and pepper as needed. Pop the yolks out of the whites and throw the yolks away. Scoop the bean mixture by the spoonful and press into the empty egg whites. Drag a fork across decoratively and sprinkle with additional paprika and the curry powder.

Low-Fat Popcorn

YIELD: 4 SERVINGS

Ingredients:

1 teaspoon (use a measuring spoon) extra virgin olive oil

Enough popcorn to cover the bottom of a saucepan

Popcorn seasoning salt

Preparation:

Heat the oil on medium high. When it begins to thin, add the popcorn and popcorn seasoning. Shake it around to coat the kernels. If you see oil in the bottom of your pan, you've used too much oil, so use less next time. Cover and turn heat down to medium. Shake continuously and occasionally lift the lid to let the steam out. If you don't let the steam out, your popcorn will be tough. Cook until there are 2–3 seconds between "pops." The key to this popcorn tasting like full-fat popcorn is the extra virgin olive oil. All other oils add fat but no flavor.

Side
Dishes

Low-Fat Onion Rings

YIELD: 4 – 6 SERVINGS

Ingredients:

2 sweet onions, cut in ¼-inch
  rings
4 egg whites
¼ teaspoon salt
¼ teaspoon pepper

¼ teaspoon garlic powder
¼ teaspoon chili powder
1 cup seasoned bread
  crumbs or crushed corn
  flakes

Cooking Instructions:

Preheat oven to 375 degrees. Separate the onion rings. Beat the egg whites with the seasoning ingredients. Dip the rings into the egg whites and dredge in the bread crumbs or corn flakes. Bake on a baking sheet lined with parchment paper for 15 minutes or until crisp.

Rice and Beans

YIELD: 6 SERVINGS

Ingredients:

1 can red kidney beans
1½ cups rice
1 onion, minced
3 cloves garlic, minced
1 bay leaf

1 teaspoon thyme or 2 sprigs
of fresh thyme
1 fresh hot pepper, seeded
and chopped

Cooking Instructions:

Drain the beans and reserve the liquid. Measure the liquid and add enough water to make 3 cups. Place the liquid, and beans, rice, and spices in a saucepan. Bring to a boil, and let boil 5 minutes. Cover and lower the heat to low. Let cook undisturbed for 20 minutes for white rice, 45 to 50 minutes for brown rice. Remove bay leaf before serving.

Mashed Potatoes

YIELD: 4 SERVINGS

Ingredients:

4 russet potatoes
4 chicken bouillon cubes
1 cup skim milk or fat-free
   buttermilk or fat-free
   sour cream

1 package butter substitute
   such as Butter Buds®
1 teaspoon garlic or onion
   powder
Salt and pepper to taste

Cooking Instructions:

Clean potatoes well. Cut up and place in a saucepan with cold water and bouillon cubes. Boil potatoes until tender. Drain. Add the Butter Buds®, garlic or onion powder, salt and pepper. Mash with a fork or potato masher. Add skim milk as needed to obtain desired texture and smoothness.

Swiss Onion Rice

YIELD: 3 – 4 SERVINGS

Ingredients:

Broth for sautéeing
1 medium onion, finely
chopped (or ¾ cup)
1 cup rice

1½ cups broth, beef or
chicken, defatted
½ cup white wine
1 cup mushrooms, sliced

Cooking Instructions:

In a saucepan over high heat, add about a tablespoon of broth, let brown, and evaporate. Add a tablespoon more and swirl around. Sauté the onion and rice until golden brown. Add liquids and mushrooms. Bring to a boil. Cover, reduce heat to low, and simmer for 25 minutes for white rice, 45 to 50 minutes for brown rice. To obtain desired flavor, you may combine the wine and broth in various quantities as long as you maintain a total of 2 cups of liquid.

Nonfat Buttered Rice

YIELD: 3 – 4 SERVINGS

Ingredients:

4 cups defatted chicken
   broth
2 cups white rice
1 onion, minced

½ package Butter Buds® or
   similar nonfat butter
   substitute

Cooking Instructions:

Bring the broth, rice, and onion to a boil in a medium saucepan. Cover and reduce heat. Cook for 20 minutes. Remove from heat and stir in butter substitute.

Burgers and Sandwiches

Burgers

YIELD: 4 SERVINGS

Ingredients:

1½ pounds 95% lean
  ground beef or ground
  turkey breast or
  combination of both

1 package onion soup mix
½ cup quick cooking oats
Pepper and garlic powder

Cooking Instructions:

Mix ingredients together. Divide in half. Divide in half again. Shape into 4 patties. Grill or pan-fry over medium heat.

C.B.L.T. (Canadian Bacon, Lettuce, and Tomato) Sandwich

2 slices Canadian bacon
Leaf lettuce
2 slices tomato

1 tablespoon fat-free
  mayonnaise
2 slices whole wheat bread

Nacho Sandwich

¼ cup fat-free refried beans
1 slice fat-free cheddar
  cheese
4–6 jalapeño slices

1 onion slice
2 slices whole wheat or white
  bread

Smoked Turkey Rueben Sandwich

1 tablespoon fat-free
  Thousand Island
  dressing
2–3 tablespoons sauerkraut

¼ pound smoked turkey
1 slice fat-free Swiss cheese
2 slices pumpernickel or
  marble rye

PIZZAS

Begin with a fat-free crust. You can make it using a pizza dough recipe or buy one at the grocery store. Be creative. If you can't find a crust specifically made for pizza, try something like pita bread. You can make your own tomato sauce or buy one of the fat-free sauces that comes in a jar and spice it up with a little extra basil, oregano, crushed red pepper, and garlic.

Barbeque Pizza

Ingredients:

Barbeque sauce
Grated fat-free cheddar cheese
Sliced grilled chicken

Thinly sliced or chopped onion
Jalapeños (optional)

Cooking Instructions:

Pour barbeque sauce on your crust. Add remaining ingredients. Broil or bake at 400 degrees for about 8 minutes, or until the cheese melts.

Mexican Pizza

Ingredients:

Fat-free refried beans
Seasoned ground meat (lean beef, chicken, or turkey). There are excellent taco meat seasoning mixes at your grocery store.

Grated fat-free cheddar or Monterey Jack cheese
Chopped lettuce
Chopped tomatoes
Diced onion
Fat-free sour cream and salsa or picante sauce

Cooking Instructions:

Spread fat-free refried beans on your crust. Add remaining ingredients. Broil or bake at 400 degrees for about 8 minutes, or until the cheese melts.

Oriental Pizza

Ingredients:

Plum or hoisin sauce
Shrimp or shredded chicken
  (you can marinate it in
  a mixture of soy, ginger,
  and garlic)

Shredded raw cabbage
Shredded carrots
Chopped green onion

Cooking Instructions:

Spread plum or hoisin sauce on your crust. Add remaining ingredients. Broil or bake at 400 degrees for about 8 minutes.

Classic Vegetable Pizza

Ingredients:

Tomato sauce
Fat-free mozzarella cheese,
  grated

Sliced mushrooms
Diced green pepper
Diced onion

Cooking Instructions:

Spread tomato sauce on your crust. Add remaining ingredients. Bake or broil at 400 degrees for about 8 minutes or until cheese melts.

Breakfast Pizza

Ingredients:

Egg whites
Smoked turkey breast

Grated fat-free cheddar
cheese
Diced green onion

Cooking Instructions:

Scramble egg whites, then spread them on your crust (whole wheat crust would be a good choice). Add remaining ingredients. Bake or broil at 400 degrees for about 8 minutes or until cheese melts.

Middle Eastern Pizza

Ingredients:

Fat-free hummus
Diced tomatoes

Chopped parsley
Ground cumin

Cooking Instructions:

Spread fat-free hummus on your crust. Add remaining ingredients. Bake or broil at 400 degrees for about 8 minutes.

Casseroles
and Stews

Pizza Casserole

YIELD: 4 – 6 SERVINGS

Ingredients:

1 pound lean ground sirloin or 90–95% lean ground beef
1 large onion, chopped
2 garlic cloves, minced
1 green pepper, chopped
8 ounces sliced mushrooms
28 ounces spaghetti or pizza sauce
2 teaspoons Italian herb seasoning
½ teaspoon crushed red pepper
1 pound fettuccine, cooked according to package instructions
1 cup grated fat-free mozzarella cheese
½ cup fat-free Parmesan cheese

Cooking Instructions:

Preheat oven to 350 degrees. Brown ground meat in skillet. Place browned meat in a colander and rinse under hot water to remove any excess fat drippings, then drain. In a large saucepan brown onion and garlic. Add green peppers, mushrooms, ground meat, spaghetti sauce, and seasonings. Cook for about 10 minutes. Add a little water if sauce is too thick. Stir to mix. Add fettuccine. Place mixture in a large casserole, sprinkle with cheese, and bake 20 minutes until bubbly.

Taco Casserole

YIELD: 4 SERVINGS

Ingredients:

3 cups rice
1½ pounds 90% lean or better ground meat, cooked
1 onion, chopped
2 16-ounce cans diced tomatoes
1 bell pepper, chopped
1 pound corn

1 package taco mix
1 cup cheddar cheese, grated
2 cans pinto beans
1 16-ounce can stewed tomatoes
2 packages Sazon Goya (optional)
1 teaspoon cumin

Cooking Instructions:

Preheat oven to 350 degrees. Boil rice. Brown ground beef, and rinse in a colander under hot running water. Combine with the remaining ingredients. Bake for 20 minutes.

Chicken Cordon Bleu Casserole

YIELD: 4 SERVINGS

Ingredients

3½ cups chicken broth, defatted

4 boneless, skinless chicken breasts, trimmed of all fat, cut in thin strips

4 slices lean Canadian bacon or lean ham, cut in strips

1 medium onion, chopped

4 cloves garlic, chopped

2 cups rice

1 can 99% fat-free cream of chicken soup

1 pound frozen French cut green beans, thawed

1 cup fat-free Swiss cheese, shredded

Cooking Instructions:

Heat a tablespoon of broth in a large skillet on high heat. When it evaporates and begins to brown, put the meat, onion, and garlic in to brown. Add broth as needed to keep from burning. When brown, remove and set aside. In a large pot, combine the rice, remaining broth, and cream of chicken soup and bring to a boil. Stir to mix well. When it comes to a boil, add the meat-onion mixture and green beans. Cover and reduce heat. Simmer 25 minutes for white rice, 60 minutes for brown. Remove from heat, add Swiss cheese, and stir to mix well.

Chicken Broccoli Rice Casserole

YIELD: 4 – 6 SERVINGS

Ingredients:

1 pound boneless, skinless chicken breasts, trimmed of fat

Flour, salt, pepper, and garlic powder for dredging

1 large onion, chopped

4 cloves garlic, minced

Defatted chicken broth for sautéing

1 can 99% fat-free cream of mushroom soup

½ pound fresh mushrooms, sliced

Salt, pepper, and garlic powder

8 ounces grated fat-free cheese

1 pound broccoli florets

5 cups cooked rice

Cooking instructions:

Preheat oven to 350 degrees. Cut the chicken into chunks, then dredge in the flour-seasoning mixture. Brown the chicken in a large nonstick skillet. Set aside. Brown the onion and garlic in a small amount of broth, using the same skillet that has the chicken "drippings." When the onion has softened, add the cream of mushroom soup and mushrooms, and season with salt, pepper, and garlic powder to taste. Add the fat-free cheese and mix well until the sauce is a uniform color. Add fresh broccoli florets to the sauce and cook for about 5 minutes. Mix the chicken, rice, and sauce together. Put in an ovenproof casserole and bake until bubbly, about 30–40 minutes.

Rio Grande Chicken Stew

YIELD: 4 SERVINGS

Ingredients:

8 cups chicken broth, defatted

4 boneless, skinless chicken breasts, trimmed of fat, cut into bite-size pieces

4 garlic cloves, minced

1 large onion, diced

4 white rose or any potato other than russet or baking

4 carrots, cut into ½-inch rounds

1½ teaspoons ground cumin

1 teaspoon oregano, crushed

4 corn tortillas, torn into strips

2 tomatoes, chopped, or 1 can tomatoes

1 pound frozen corn

2 yellow squash, cut into ¼-inch rounds

2 zucchini, cut into ¼-inch rounds

¼ cup cilantro leaves

Cooking Instructions:

Pour 2 teaspoons of chicken both into a hot skillet. Let brown and evaporate. Add chicken chunks and brown, adding broth as necessary to keep from burning. Brown the garlic and onion. Remove and set aside. In a large stock pot, pour the remaining chicken broth, add the potatoes, carrots, cumin, oregano, and tortillas. Cover and cook for about 20 minutes on medium heat. When the potatoes and carrots are almost cooked completely, add the tomatoes, corn, squash, and zucchini. Cook for an additional 5–10 minutes, then add the cilantro. Stir to mix well.

Entrées

Fake Fried Chicken

YIELD: 4 SERVINGS

Ingredients:

4 boneless, skinless chicken breasts, trimmed of fat
16 ounces fat-free yogurt
1 cup all purpose flour
1 cup plain bread crumbs
1 cup fine bread crumbs
1 teaspoon garlic powder
1 teaspoon Italian herb seasoning
Salt and pepper
1 egg white
½ cup skim milk
Defatted chicken broth in a spray bottle

Cooking Instructions:

Preheat oven to 350 degrees. Dredge (or dip) chicken in fat-free yogurt, then roll the chicken in a combination of flour and bread crumbs. Combine all the other dry ingredients in a gallon-sized plastic zip bag. Add the chicken breasts and shake. Then beat the egg white and milk together in a bowl. Dip the breaded chicken into the egg-milk mixture. Put the chicken back into the plastic bag and shake again. Place chicken on a foil-covered cookie sheet. Mist with chicken broth until moist and bake 20–30 minutes.

Leslie's Easy Chicken

YIELD: **4** SERVINGS

Ingredients:

*4 skinless chicken breasts,
either boneless or bone-
in*
1 package onion soup mix
*3–4 baking potatoes, cut
into bite-sized pieces*

*4 carrots, cut into bite-sized
coins, or 1 cup baby
carrots*
1 medium onion, minced
4 cloves garlic, minced

Cooking Instructions:

Preheat oven to 350 degrees. Put all the ingredients
into a large zip bag and shake. Pour the mixture into
a 9x13-inch glass baking pan. Spread out and bake cov-
ered for 25 minutes. Remove the cover and bake uncov-
ered for an additional 20 minutes.

Apricot Chicken

YIELD: 4 SERVINGS

Ingredients:

4 boneless, skinless chicken breasts
1 cup apricot preserves
1 package dry onion soup mix
Salt and pepper to taste

Fat-free Russian dressing:
1 cup fat-free mayonnaise
1 tablespoon horseradish
1 teaspoon Worcestershire sauce
½ cup chili sauce or catsup
1 teaspoon grated onion

Cooking Instructions:

Preheat oven to 350 degrees. Season chicken and set aside on a foil-covered cookie sheet. Mix the remaining ingredients until blended. Pour over chicken and bake for about 30 minutes or until golden.

Chicken and Rice

YIELD: 4 SERVINGS

Ingredients:

4 boneless, skinless chicken breasts, trimmed of all fat

2 cans chicken broth, defatted

1 teaspoon chopped garlic

1 medium onion, chopped

1½ cups uncooked white or brown rice

½ teaspoon favorite herb, thyme, tarragon, or rosemary

Salt and pepper to taste

1 pound frozen peas

Cooking Instructions:

Cut the chicken into bite-sized chunks. Brown in a little bit (1–2 teaspoons) of chicken broth in a large saucepan. When browned, add the garlic and onion. Cook until they brown. Add the rice and seasoning, stirring to mix well. Combine the broth with enough water to make 3 cups. Pour into the chicken and rice mixture. Bring to a boil over high heat. Let boil a minute or two, cover, then reduce the heat to low and cook without stirring for 20 minutes for white rice or 45–50 minutes for brown rice. Add the peas, cover, and cook an additional 5–7 minutes. Stir and serve.

Most Requested Meat Loaf

YIELD: 8 SERVINGS

Ingredients:

1½ pounds lean ground beef or turkey or combination
½ cup tomato sauce or tomato juice
1 medium onion, chopped
1 bell pepper, seeded and chopped
2 egg whites
¾ cup quick or old-fashioned rolled oats
1 package onion soup mix
1 teaspoon garlic powder
Couple shakes of Worcestershire sauce
Salt and pepper
1 16-ounce can tomato basil soup

Cooking Instructions:

Preheat oven to 350 degrees. Place meat in a large bowl. Combine all other ingredients, except tomato soup, in a medium bowl and mix thoroughly. Make a well in the meat and put the contents of the medium bowl in the well. Mix well. Place a cooling rack in the middle of a foil-lined roasting pan. After putting the meat mixture into a loaf pan to shape, turn it out on the rack. Bake for 45 minutes. Top with the tomato soup and continue baking an additional 30 minutes. Let stand 10 minutes before slicing.

Pasta with Ham and Peas

YIELD: 4 SERVINGS

Ingredients:

Chicken broth for sautéing
3 garlic cloves, minced
4 green onions, chopped
½ pound lean ham or
  Canadian bacon,
  julienned
1 cup evaporated skim milk

1 package Butter Buds® or
  butter substitute
12–16 ounces fettuccine or
  your favorite pasta
1–1½ cups fresh or frozen
  peas
½ cup Parmesan cheese

Cooking Instructions:

Sauté garlic in a small amount of broth until golden. Turn heat down to low. Add the green onions and ham, and stir. Add the milk and Butter Buds®, and stir. Set aside. Cook pasta until al dente. Drain well and place pasta and peas in the pan with sauce, tossing to coat. Serve immediately with Parmesan cheese.

Shrimp Scampi

YIELD: 4 SERVINGS

Ingredients:

1 pound shrimp, shelled
1 cup defatted chicken broth
10 garlic cloves, minced
1 cup dry white wine
1 package Butter Buds® or
   butter substitute
4 cups rice, cooked
Parsley sprigs and lemon
   slices for garnish

Low-fat marinade:
3 tablespoons dry
   vermouth
2 tablespoons minced
   Italian parsley
1 teaspoon olive oil
½ teaspoon salt
Pinch of pepper

Cooking Instructions:

Mix marinade ingredients in a shallow glass bowl and marinate the shrimp for 2–3 hours. Pour several teaspoons of broth in a skillet. After the broth evaporates and browns, add the garlic and brown, then add broth as needed to keep from burning. Add the marinated shrimp and cook on medium heat until the shrimp curls. Add the white wine and Butter Buds®, then stir until the sauce thickens. Remove from heat and serve on a bed of rice. Garnish with parsley and lemon slices.

Beef and Asparagus Roll-Ups

YIELD: 4 – 6 SERVINGS AS A MAIN COURSE, 12 AS AN APPETIZER

Ingredients:

24–30 thin asparagus stalks
8 green onions
½ cup soy sauce
¼ cup sugar

Pinch of cayenne powder
1½ pounds beef tenderloin
or eye of round roast

Cooking Instructions:

Preheat broiler or grill. Rinse asparagus and cut off 4 inches from tips. Place in a shallow pan and microwave on high for 30 seconds. Cut green onions into 4-inch pieces, then julienne lengthwise. Combine soy, sugar, and cayenne in a small bowl, stirring until sugar dissolves. Slice the meat in ¼-inch slices and lightly pound each slice, individually, with a meat pounder. Dip each piece of beef in the soy mixture, and place on a baking sheet. Place one piece each of asparagus and green onion on one side of the beef and roll up. Set aside and repeat until you run out of either meat slices or vegetables. Grill or broil until slightly charred—this should take only a couple of minutes. Serve hot or room temperature.

DESSERTS

Angel Delight

YIELD: 8 SERVINGS

Ingredients:

1 angel food cake
½ cup powdered sugar
½ cup egg substitute
1 teaspoon almond extract
   or 1½ teaspoons vanilla
   extract

12-ounce carton fat-free
   whipped topping
6 hard, sugar-free caramel
   candies, crushed

Preparation:

Slice the angel food cake and cover the bottom of a 9x13-inch glass baking dish. Combine sugar, egg substitute, and flavoring and fold into whipped topping. Layer angel food slices with whipped topping. Sprinkle the crushed candies on top. Cover with plastic wrap and freeze. Serve frozen.

Banana Pudding

YIELD: 10 – 12 SERVINGS

Ingredients:

1 8-ounce package fat-free cream cheese, softened

1 14-ounce can fat-free, sweetened condensed milk

2 cups skim milk

1 6-ounce package instant vanilla pudding

8 ounces fat-free whipped topping

4 bananas, sliced

1 12-ounce package reduced fat vanilla wafers

Preparation:

With beaters, cream the cheese until smooth. Mix in the next three ingredients. Fold in half of the whipped topping. Layer the pudding, cookies, and bananas in a glass or ceramic dish. Top with remaining topping. Chill.

Strawberry Cheesecake Dream

YIELD: 6 – 8 SERVINGS

Ingredients:

1 pound frozen strawberries
2 packages strawberry
  gelatin dessert mix

12 ounces (one can) very cold
  strawberry soda (regular
  or diet)
8 ounces fat-free cream
  cheese, softened

Preparation:

Defrost strawberries, then heat in a medium saucepan until softened. With a slotted spoon remove and set aside. Add enough water to strawberry juice to make 2 cups. Bring to a boil. Remove from heat. Add gelatin. Stir until dissolved. Add strawberry soda and chill for 4 hours. One hour before the gelatin has set, take the cream cheese out of refrigerator to soften. When the gelatin has chilled for 4 hours, remove from the refrigerator. With an electric mixer beat the cream cheese until smooth. Scoop into the gelatin mixture and beat until all the cream cheese is blended evenly. Stir in the fruit, pour into a mold, and chill 6 hours or overnight.

Key Lime Pie

YIELD: 8 SERVINGS

Ingredients:

*1 14-ounce can fat-free
   sweetened condensed
   milk*
*Egg Beaters®, equivalent to
   2 eggs*
3–4 ounces lime juice

*1 tablespoon Grand
   Marnier (optional)*
*1 low-fat graham cracker
   crust*
Fat-free whipped topping

Cooking Instructions:

Combine sweetened condensed milk and Egg Beaters®—try not to add too much air. Slowly add lime juice and Grand Marnier. Mix until well blended. Pour into pie crust and bake at 350 degrees for 12–15 minutes. Top with fat-free whipped topping.

Banana Parfait Pie

YIELD: 6 – 8 SERVINGS

Ingredients:

4 ripe bananas
1 low-fat graham cracker
  crust
1 12-ounce carton fat-free
  whipped topping

2 ounces peanut brittle (the
  inexpensive kind that's
  mostly sugar and very few
  peanuts) or 6 hard
  caramel candies
Fat-free caramel sauce

Preparation:

Cut the bananas into ¼-inch slices. Line the pie crust with banana slices. Spread a couple of heaping scoops of whipped topping over slices then sprinkle half of candy on top. Repeat the process two more times, drizzling the fat-free caramel sauce on top of the last layer instead of candy. Freeze for 4 hours or overnight. Serve frozen.

C H A P T E R
10

The Slimdown for Life Guide to Eating Out

Before you go out and start special ordering, make sure you know what you're talking about. It's a little counter-productive to go into an Italian restaurant and order a steaming plate of a creamy pasta dish such as fettucine Alfredo and say, "And make that low fat." No chef can take the cream out of creamy pasta. The waiter will respect your request more if you ask for pasta dressed only in tomato, basil, and garlic, or perhaps with a little wine.

Here's another common mistake: You sit down for breakfast in a restaurant and proudly ask for an egg white omelette. But you don't specify how you want it prepared. Yes, you will get your egg whites, all right, but the omelette may be swimming in butter and cov-ered with cheese. You end up with an omelette that has

254 LARRY NORTH'S SLIMDOWN FOR LIFE

thirty grams of fat! The lesson? Be specific. If you ask for an egg white omelette without cheese and prepared with no butter or oil, then you have just brought the fat content of that omelette down to almost zero. Don't simply ask for grilled chicken. When you order fish or chicken, ask for it to be cooked with lemon or lime juice as an alternative to oil or butter. You will never feel worse than when you order what you think is a low-fat piece of grilled chicken and learn later that it is swamped with fat, all because the cook added four to five tablespoons of cooking oil. You have to specify!

Finally, if you're at a restaurant or bakery and you see certain claims about how many calories are in one of their dishes, be careful. I'll never forget how a New York magazine once did a nutritional analysis of twenty bagels bought at a variety of shops around New York City. Although the bagels were advertised as being around 200 calories each, the magazine discovered that the average calorie count was more than twice that! The lowest-calorie bagel had 307 calories and the highest-calorie one had an amazing 552 calories! Don't necessarily trust a restaurant or bakery when it tells you on the menu how many calories are in one of its dishes. The magazine found one bakery advertising a fat-free muffin. When analyzed, the muffin contained 750 calories and forty-five grams of fat. The baker later explained away his false advertising by saying, "I didn't want the people feeling guilty about eating my food!"

A restaurant might claim on the menu that its food has only a certain number of calories, but I wouldn't accept those claims on face value. It's one thing for the restaurateur to put down some calorie counts on the menu. It's another thing entirely for the kitchen staff to try to follow those caloric guidelines. I've been in the back of a lot of kitchens where oils were being doused everywhere on all kinds of food. That same New York magazine went to various pizza parlors and Italian restaurants and discovered the average pizza slice had twice as many calories and three times as much fat as advertised. In fact, one restaurant advertised a "healthy" slice of pizza that had 610 calories, and seventeen grams of fat. One slice!

Specific Restaurant Choices

Here are some specific dishes you can look for, regardless which restaurant you visit.

French: You can ask for an egg white omelette, fillet of sole, poached sea bass, trout, bay scallops, or other grilled fish or white meat in wine sauce. There's usually a standard salad you can get without dressing. If it's a spinach salad, ask that no bacon or egg be added. Avoid Hollandaise or any cream-based sauce as well as sautéed dishes unless they are sautéed in water. Avoid high-fat dishes such as duck, pâté de fois gras.

Italian: Look for a vegetable plate with no sauce, meatless pasta with oil-free marinara or wine sauce, or a vegetarian pizza with no cheese and an oil-free crust. Avoid any cream sauces and fatty meats such as prosciutto, Parmesan cheese, breaded veal, breaded vegetables, and white breads. Also watch out for olive oil, which many restaurants tend to overuse. Plain pasta might seem like a good choice, but it often contains oil from the boiling pot. One of my favorite Italian meals consists of grilled portabello mushrooms with balsamic vinegar, grilled chicken Caesar salad with no croutons, dressing on the side, and a small bowl of plain pasta with marinara sauce on the side.

Mexican: Look for fresh fish or chicken breast marinated in lime juice with beans and rice. You can also order unfried corn tortillas, chicken enchiladas without the cheese or cream sauce, or chicken fajitas grilled in lemon or lime juice instead of oil. Avoid cheese, chips, sour cream, guacamole, and refried beans (ask for whole beans instead). It's easy to make a North Plate at a Mexican restaurant: Just order grilled chicken fajitas with no oil, corn tortillas (instead of higher-fat flour tortillas), rice instead of refried beans, pico de gallo instead of guacamole, and no cheese. Have the lettuce, onion, and tomato on the side. If you see spinach enchiladas on the menu, you can ask for a side of spinach as your fibrous vegetable.

Chinese: Go for Moo Goo Gai Pan without sauce. Ask for fresh or steamed fish and vegetables. Make sure only white meat chicken is used in dishes. Ask that the dishes be stir-fried in broth or water instead of oil or salt. Choose the dishes that come with sliced meat rather than diced meat because diced meat is often from fatty cuts. Order steamed rice instead of fried rice. Avoid egg rolls, any batter-fried item, any egg dishes, and dishes loaded with nuts. Don't order beef or pork, and never order duck (an average three-and-a-half-ounce serving of Peking duck has thirty grams of fat).

Vietnamese, Thai, or Japanese: These restaurants are great for the North Program, because they use very little oil in their cooking to begin with. You can order any type of dish with no egg and no oil, and it's likely to be low fat. You can also order a spring roll that's like an egg roll, except make sure it is not fried. Japanese restaurants also cook many items without oil or margarine. Sushi places can be ideal for your program, as long as you order the less-fattening items on the menu. I recommend the California roll minus avocado or mayonnaise. However, be careful because some sushi can be extremely high in fat, such as eel and ahi tuna, and of course anything that is fried.

Steak house: At a steak restaurant, ask for a large dinner salad without cheese or croutons, and ask for a baked potato with yogurt or Dijon mustard. Most of these restaurants offer grilled chicken on the menu. If you order it, ask that all fat be trimmed and no oil be used in preparation. You usually can have shrimp or perhaps lobster. But if you want to eat steak, then order one. My suggestion is to get a smaller cut of filet (six ounces is a good size) and have the chef butterfly it on the grill, in which he cuts it down the middle (which helps get rid of some fat in the grilling process).

Fast food: There is very little nutritional value in fast food. It hits you with a horde of calories that are basically sugar and fat without any fiber or vitamins. Don't be fooled into thinking that fast-food chicken is better than hamburgers. A single fried chicken nugget contains an entire tablespoon of mostly saturated fat. Fast-food chicken sandwiches have as much fat as hamburgers. As for fried chicken, the original healthful piece is so soaked in oil that the fat has seeped down to the bone. If you must eat at a fast-food restaurant, try to go vegetarian. Get the lettuce and tomato and look for a baked potato.

Pizza place: At a pizza restaurant, order a pizza with peppers, mushrooms, onions, shrimp, and chicken if available—and no cheese. That alone saves you a tremendous number of calories. Sometimes you can add extra sauce.

American chain restaurants: Actually, these restaurants have become very accessible for North eaters. Most of them carry grilled chicken, grilled shrimp, brown rice, black beans, salads, fat-free dressing, and steamed vegetables.

Cafeterias: Again, at cafeterias, turn vegeterian. Most of the meats offered at cafeterias are soaked in oil or butter, as are the vegetables. Your safest choices are going to be straight dinner salads with dressing on the side. Avoid all casseroles, and ask how the vegetables have been cooked.

Greasy spoon: You can even follow the North Program here. If you're eating breakfast, try five to seven hard-boiled or poached eggs with the yolks removed, a bowl of oatmeal, and dry toast. You can special order a grilled white meat item and vegetables that are not sautéed, fried, or buttered.

11

The Sixty-Second Workouts

The Sixty-Second Workouts are broken down into four categories—Upper Body, Lower Body, Abdominals, and Stretches. Each exercise should take no more than sixty seconds. I'm not particularly concerned about you trying to work out your various body parts equally. Divide them however you want—but do try to get in some stretches and abdominal work each day.

Here's a secret about performing your Sixty-Second Workouts. You can build plenty of muscle using little or no weight if you have the right form. The amount of weight you're moving is never the measure of your success. It's form. And the secret to ensuring good form is posture. In life, you don't have to walk around as if you're a Marine standing at attention. But you do in the Sixty-Second Workouts. Correct posture in almost every one of these exercises means your back stays straight, your shoulders stay back, your chest sticks out, and your legs remain straight but not locked in position. If you find your shoulders slumping, your back rounding off, your hips thrusting forward, or your back jerking, then you are not working the muscle as well as you could.

As you begin, the pace of your reps is also very important. (Each time you do a single movement, such as going up on your toes and down, it's called a rep—for repetition.) Slow your reps down. Try for rhythmic consistency. The key word to remember is control. You must control your body. If you are losing control of the movement, you are doing it too fast. That's why, after the first several reps of an exercise, you should feel the muscle working. If you don't, you are doing your reps too quickly.

Although I want you to start off slowly and not over-work yourself, start thinking of ways to use Sixty-Second Workouts during idle moments in your day. You can do Modified Push-ups, for example, against the kitchen counter if you happen to be waiting for something to cook on the stove. Or you can do your extra Toe Raises while talking on the telephone. That is the point of Sixty-Second Workouts. You can do them almost anywhere at any time of the day.

Upper Body

Front Shoulder Raise

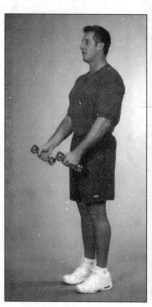 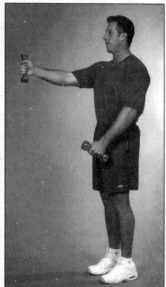

Instructions:

1. Stand with your knees and hips slightly bent to create a slight forward tilt with the upper body.

2. Keep your back straight and shoulders back.

3. Start with your arms in front of the body, elbows slightly bent and thumbs facing forward.

4. Raise your arms up to about shoulder height, keeping the elbows slightly bent and the dumbbells parallel to the body.

5. Lower the arms back down slowly and repeat.

Tips:

1. Keep the knees slightly bent and back straight.

2. Avoid twisting or rotating the arms.

3. Keep the elbows slightly bent and maintain a loose grip on the dumbbells.

Side Shoulder Raise

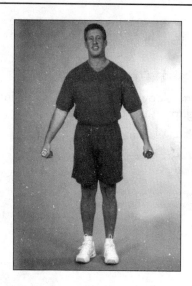

Instructions:

1. Stand up straight with your knees and hips slightly bent to create a slight forward tilt with the upper body.

2. Keep your back straight and shoulders back.

3. Start with your arms out to the side of the body, elbows slightly bent and thumbs facing forward.

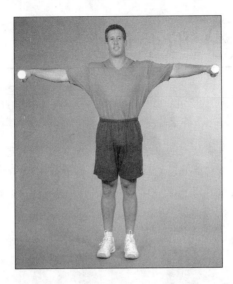

4. Raise your arms out to just below shoulder height, keeping the elbows slightly bent and the dumbbells level.

5. Lower them back down slowly, then repeat.

Tips:

1. Keep the knees slightly bent and back straight.

2. Avoid twisting or rotating the arms.

3. Keep the elbows slightly bent and maintain a loose grip on the dumbbells.

Bicep Curl

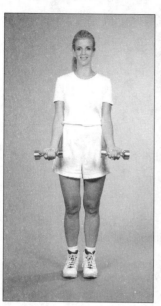 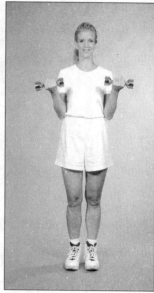

Instructions:

1. Stand up straight with your knees and hips slightly bent to create a slight forward tilt with the upper body.

2. Keep your back straight and shoulders back.

3. Start with your arms straight down and to the sides of the body with your elbows slightly bent.

4. Raise your lower arms and dumbbells up as far as possible without moving your shoulders or upper arms.

5. Hold, squeeze the biceps, then slowly lower them back down and repeat.

Tips:

1. Keep the knees slightly bent and back straight.

2. Avoid locking the elbows at the bottom.

3. Keep the elbows in place and maintain a loose grip on the dumbbells.

Modified Push-ups

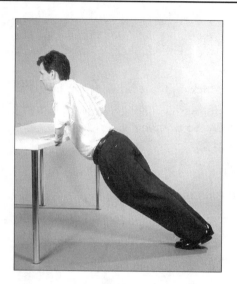

Instructions:

1. Lean against a desk, table, or any solid object that will not slide or move under your weight.

2. Place your hands outside your shoulders by approximately 8 to 12 inches. (The distance is determined by the length of your upper arm or the distance from your elbow to shoulder.)

3. Start with your arms and back straight and your ankles only slightly bent.

4. Keeping your back straight and your legs stiff, lower your body down until your elbows are bent about 90 degrees.

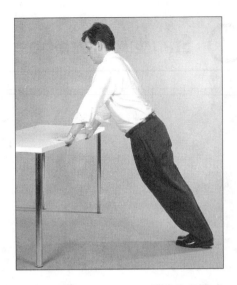

5. Hold, then slowly push your body back up to the starting position and repeat.

Tips:

1. Keep the back straight and avoid allowing the spine to sway or round at any time.

2. Avoid excessive bending of the ankles and wrists.

3. Go slowly and try to keep from bending the elbows more than 90 degrees at the bottom or locking them out at the top.

Standard Push-ups

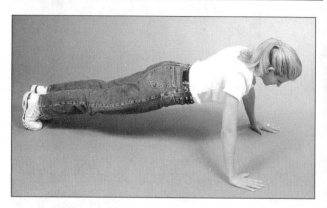

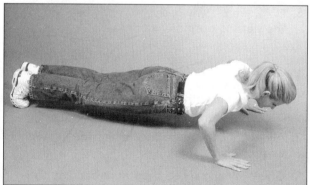

Instructions:

1. Get on the floor, facedown, with your weight supported by your flexed wrists and toes. Place your hands outside your shoulders by approximately 8 to 12 inches. (The distance

is determined by the length of your upper arm or the distance from your elbow to shoulder.)

2. Straighten your legs and arms. Keep your hands slightly above the shoulder as well as outside of them.

3. Start with your arms and back straight and your ankles only slightly bent.

4. Keeping your back straight and your legs stiff, lower your body down until your elbows are bent about 90 degrees.

5. Hold, then slowly push your body back up to the starting position and repeat.

Tips:

1. Keep the back straight and avoid allowing the spine to sway or round at any time.

2. Avoid excessive bending of the ankles and wrists.

3. Go slowly and try to keep from bending the elbows more than 90 degrees at the bottom or locking them out at the top.

Bent Knee Push-ups

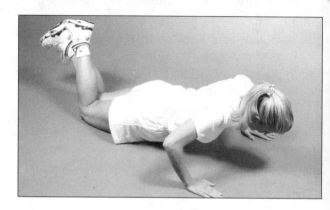

Instructions:

1. Get on the floor, facedown, with your knees bent and your weight supported by your flexed wrists. Place your hands outside your shoulders by approximately 8 to 12 inches. (The distance is determined by the length of your upper arm or the distance from your elbow to shoulder.)

2. Keeping your knees bent, cross one foot over the other, and straighten your body so that your hands are now slightly above the shoulder as well as outside of them.

3. Start with your arms and back straight.

4. Keeping your back straight and your knees bent, lower your body down until your elbows are bent about 90 degrees.

5. Hold, then slowly push your body back up to the starting position and repeat.

Tips:

1. Keep the back straight and avoid allowing the spine to sway or round at any time.

2. Avoid allowing the knees to slide on the floor.

3. Go slowly and try to keep from bending the elbows more than 90 degrees at the bottom or locking them out at the top.

One-Arm Dumbell Row

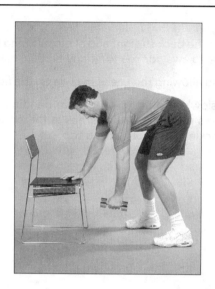

Instructions:

1. Spread your feet well outside the shoulders and place one hand on a chair, desk, table, or any solid object that will not slide under your weight.

2. Bend your knees and straighten your back.

3. Start with the other arm straight down from the shoulder with the elbow pointed back and slightly bent.

4. Keeping your back straight and your knees bent, pull your arm and the dumbbell up until your elbow is bent about 90 degrees.

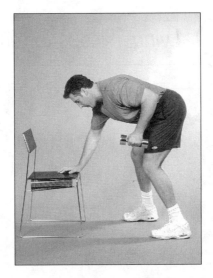

5. Hold, squeeze the back muscles, then slowly lower the arm and dumbbell back to the starting position and repeat.

Tips:

1. Keep the back and neck straight and avoid allowing the spine to sway or round at any time.

2. Keep the elbow pointed back and close to the side throughout the exercise.

3. Go slowly and try to keep from bending the elbow more than 90 degrees at the top or locking it out at the top.

Lying Triceps Extension

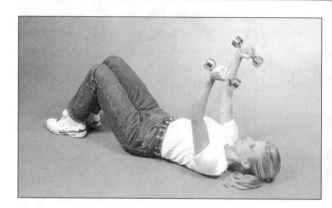

Instructions:

1. Lie comfortably on your back on the floor with the knees bent.

2. Start with the arms straight up from the shoulders with the elbows and dumbbells parallel to the body.

3. Keeping the elbow directly over the shoulder, slowly lower the upper arm and dumbbell until the elbow is bent approximately 90 degrees.

4. Hold, then slowly pull your arms and the dumbbells back up to their starting position and repeat.

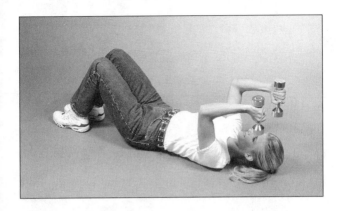

Tips:

1. Keep the shoulders down and in place throughout the exercise.

2. Avoid bending the elbows any more than 90 degrees at the bottom or locking them out at the top.

3. Lift slowly and keep the dumbbells parallel to the body throughout the exercise.

Lower Body

Leg Raise

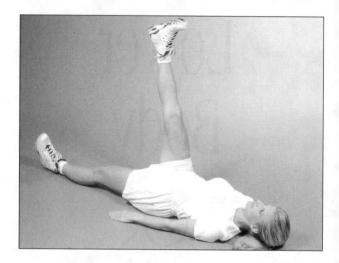

Instructions:

1. Lie comfortably on your back on the floor with one leg straight up.

2. Carefully pull the leg toward your head, stretching the hamstring.

3. Tighten your abdominal muscles, flatten the back, and slowly begin lowering the leg down.

4. Lower the leg down only as far as you can while keeping the back flat.

5. Hold, then slowly pull the leg back up and stretch the hamstring.

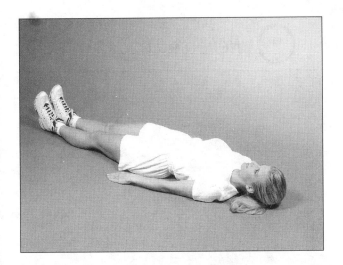

Tips:

1. Try to keep tension on the abdominal muscles and back flat throughout the exercise. (Remember that this is an abdominal exercise as well as a hamstring stretch.)

2. Do not begin with the leg on the floor and do not lower down any farther than you are able to keep the back flat.

3. Lift and stretch slowly and try to breathe out as you lift the leg.

Reverse Lunge

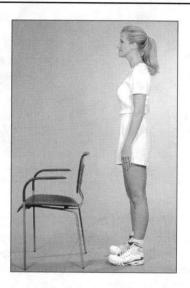

Instructions:

1. Stand with your knees and hips slightly bent.

2. Start with your weight primarily shifted to one leg and centered over the ankle.

3. Keeping the back straight, step back with the other leg and plant the toe firmly against the ground with the knee only slightly bent.

4. Hold, balance, then return to your starting position, keeping your back straight and your weight over the ankle of the lead leg. Repeat.

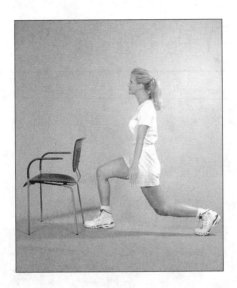

Tips:

1. Keep the back straight throughout the exercise.

2. Avoid having the knee of the lead leg push over the toe, or excessively bending the back knee.

3. Keep the weight over the ankle of the lead leg, and focus on keeping tension on the buttocks muscle of the lead leg.

Heel Presses

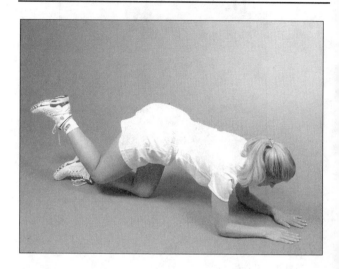

Instructions:

1. Position yourself comfortably on the floor on all fours with the back and neck straight.

2. Start with one leg slightly off the floor and the knee bent at approximately 90 degrees.

3. Slowly lift the leg while keeping the back and neck straight.

4. Focus on squeezing the buttock muscle on the same leg you are lifting.

5. Hold, then slowly lower the leg back to the starting position. Repeat.

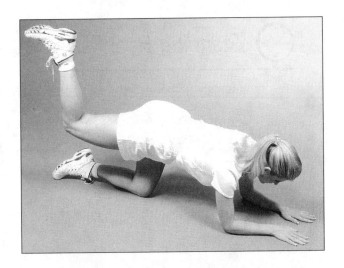

Tips:

1. Keep the back and neck straight throughout the exercise.

2. Avoid lifting the leg to a point where you feel any discomfort in the lower back.

3. Lift slowly and try to keep tension in the buttocks muscle.

Standing Heel Raise

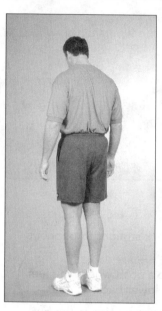 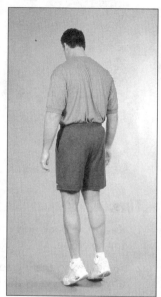

Instructions:

1. Stand with your feet under your hips, knees very slightly bent, and toes pointed straight ahead.

2. Lean slightly forward and balance against the wall, table, desk, or any stable object.

3. Begin with your heels slightly off the ground.

4. Raise your body up as far as possible and hold.

5. Lower your body slowly down and repeat.

Tips:

1. Avoid straightening or further bending of the knees once set.

2. Go slowly and avoid bouncing.

3. Try to keep the ankles from rolling out or in during this exercise.

Standing Single Heel Raise

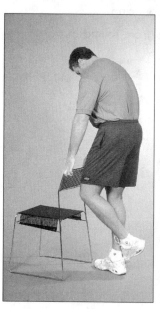 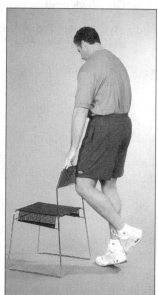

Instructions:

1. Stand on one leg with the foot aligned directly under your body, the knee bent very slightly and the toe pointed straight ahead. Bend the other leg, and cross your ankles.

2. Lean slightly forward and balance against the wall, table, desk, or any stable object.

3. Begin with the heel of your supporting leg slightly off the ground.

4. Raise your body up as far as possible and hold.

5. Lower your body slowly down and repeat.

Tips:

1. Avoid straightening or further bending of the knee once set.

2. Go slowly and avoid bouncing.

3. Try to keep the ankle from rolling out or in during this exercise.

Seated Resisted Heel Raise

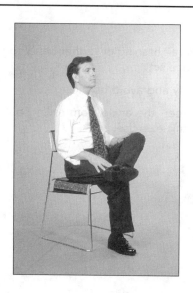

Instructions:

1. Sit up straight with your feet pointed forward and your knees bent about 90 degrees.

2. Place left ankle on right knee as shown.

3. Raise right heel slowly and hold.

4. Lower right heel slowly to floor.

5. Repeat steps 1–4 for sixty seconds.

6. Repeat steps 1–5 for left heel.

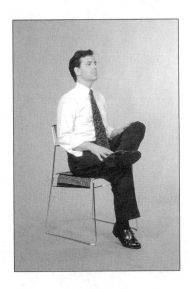

Tips:

1. Keep good posture throughout the exercise.

2. Go slowly and avoid bouncing.

3. Try to keep your ankles from rolling out or in during this exercise.

Abdominals

Crunches

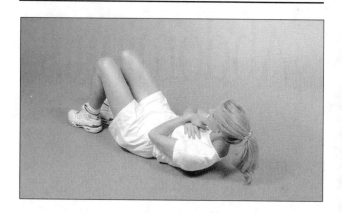

Instructions:

1. Lie comfortably on your back on the floor with your arms crossed over the chest and your knees bent.

2. Start with your head and shoulders off the ground, press your lower back firmly against the floor, and tighten your abdominals.

3. Begin breathing out and slowly pull your rib cage toward your pelvis as far as you are able.

4. Breathe out any remaining air, hold, then slowly lower your rib cage down to the starting position while breathing in. Repeat.

Tips:

1. Keep the lower back pressed firmly against the floor and maintain constant tension in the abdominal muscles throughout the exercise.

2. Keep the chin slightly tucked and avoid moving the head independently.

3. Lift slowly and breathe properly throughout the exercise.

Chair Sit-ups

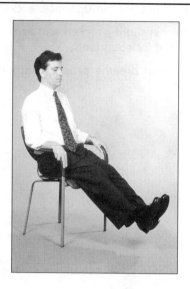

Instructions:

1. Sit back in a chair and hold on firmly to the seat or arms of the chair. Keep your legs together.

2. Extend legs slightly and lift slightly off the ground.

3. Raise your knees slowly toward your chest, breathe out, and contract your abdominals.

4. Lower your knees slowly down, while breathing in until your legs are in the original extended position.

5. Repeat steps 3–4 for sixty seconds.

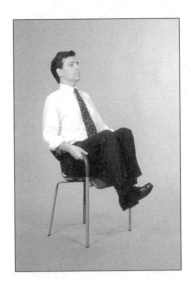

Tips:

1. Avoid straightening or arching the back.

2. Be sure to breathe out as you raise the knees and are contracting the abdominal muscles. Breathe in as you lower the legs.

3. Go slowly and try to keep constant tension in the abdominals.

Stretches

Full Body Stretch

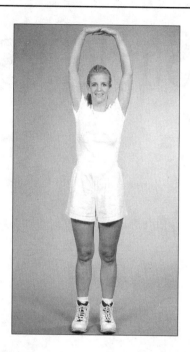

Instructions:

1. Stand up straight with the knees and hips slightly bent.

2. Keeping your back straight, reach up with both arms and interlock the fingers.

3. Slowly straighten the arms and elevate the shoulders as high as possible.

4. Hold for 8 to 12 seconds, relax, then repeat.

Tips:

1. Maintain good posture and avoid twisting the back or neck.

2. Allow the fingers to relax and separate as the arms straighten.

3. Stretch slowly and try to breathe out as you stretch.

Abdominal and Hips Flexor Stretch for Hips

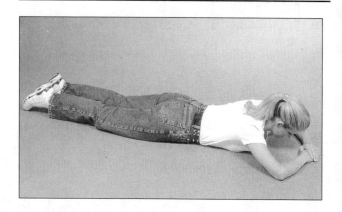

Instructions:

1. Lie comfortably facedown on the floor with the upper body supported by the elbows.

2. Slowly pull your lower leg toward your buttocks.

3. Slowly attempt to lift the knee up and off the floor.

4. Hold for 8 to 12 seconds, relax, then repeat.

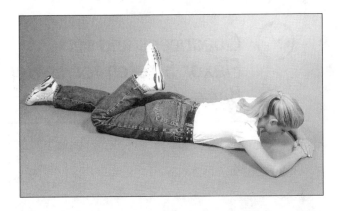

Tips:

1. If you have a history of lower back pain, check with your physician before performing this exercise.

2. Avoid lifting the knee to a point where you feel any discomfort in the lower back.

3. Stretch slowly and try to breathe out as you stretch.

Quadriceps and Hip Flexor Stretch for Lower Back

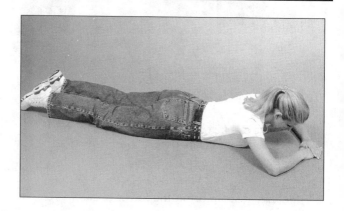

Instructions:

1. Lie comfortably facedown on the floor with the upper body supported by the elbows.

2. Slowly pull your rib cage up and forward until you feel a stretch in your hip flexors and abdominal region.

3. Hold for 8 to 12 seconds, relax, then repeat.

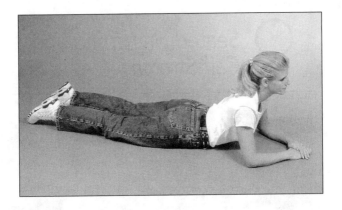

Tips:

1. If you have a history of lower back pain, check with your physician before performing this exercise.

2. Avoid lifting the rib cage to a point where you feel any discomfort in the lower back.

3. Stretch slowly and try to breathe out as you stretch.

Seated Hamstring and Calf Stretch

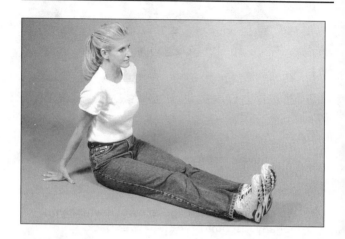

Instructions:

1. Sit comfortably on the floor with legs straight out and arms behind you, with palms resting on the floor.

2. Slowly attempt to straighten the spine and feel the hamstrings stretch.

3. Then slowly pull the toes back until you feel your calves stretch.

4. Hold for 8 to 12 seconds, relax, then repeat.

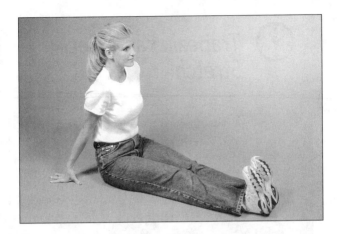

Tips:

1. Maintain good posture and avoid twisting or rounding the back or spine.

2. If you are unable to straighten your back with the knees straight, then perform this exercise while sitting on a low bench, footstool, or perhaps a briefcase.

3. Stretch slowly and try to breathe out as you stretch.

Trapezius and Neck Stretch

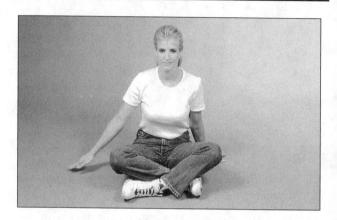

Instructions:

1. Stand or sit comfortably.

2. Keeping your back straight, slowly reach down and out from your body with one arm as far as possible while slightly leaning your head to the opposite side.

3. Hold for 8 to 12 seconds, relax, then repeat or stretch the other side.

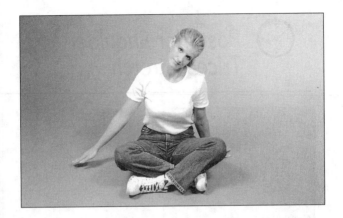

Tips:

1. Maintain good posture and avoid twisting the back or spine.

2. Pull the head slightly forward when leaning it to the side.

3. Stretch slowly and try to breathe out as you stretch.

Posterior Shoulder and Tricep Stretch

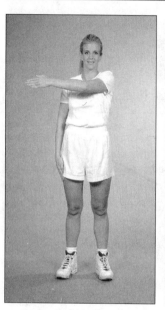 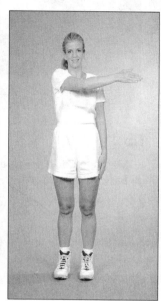

Instructions:

1. Stand up straight with the knees and hips slightly bent.

2. Keeping your back straight, slowly reach across your body with one arm as far as possible.

3. Hold for 8 to 12 seconds, relax, then repeat or stretch the other arm.

Tips:

1. Maintain good posture and avoid twisting the back or neck.

2. Keep the elbow pointed out away from the body throughout the exercise.

3. Stretch slowly and try to breathe out as you stretch.

Metric Conversion Chart

Formulas for conversion:

Fahrenheit to Celsius: Subtract 32, multiply by 5, then divide by 9.

For example:

$$212°F - 32 = 180$$
$$180 \times 5 = 900$$
$$900 \div 9 = 100°C$$

Celsius to Fahrenheit: Multiply by 9, divide by 5, then add 32.

For example:

$$100°C \times 9 = 900$$
$$900 \div 5 = 180$$
$$180 + 32 = 212°F$$

Temperatures (Fahrenheit to Celsius)

−10°F =	−23°C	coldest part of freezer
0°F =	−17°C	freezer
32°F =	0°C	water freezes
68°F =	20°C	room temperature
85°F =	29°C	
100°F =	38°C	

Temperatures (Fahrenheit to Celsius) (*cont.*)

115°F =	46°C	water simmers
135°F =	57°C	water scalds
140°F =	60°C	
150°F =	66°C	
160°F =	71°C	
170°F =	77°C	
180°F =	82°C	
190°F =	88°C	
200°F =	95°C	
205°F =	96°C	
212°F =	100°C	water boils, at sea level
225°F =	110°C	
250°F =	120°C	very low (or slow) oven
275°F =	135°C	very low (or slow) oven
300°F =	150°C	low (or slow) oven
325°F =	165°C	low (or moderately slow) oven
350°F =	180°C	moderate oven
375°F =	190°C	moderate (or moderately hot) oven
400°F =	205°C	hot oven
425°F =	220°C	hot oven
450°F =	230°C	very hot oven
475°F =	245°C	very hot oven
500°F =	260°C	extremely hot oven/broiling
525°F =	275°C	extremely hot oven/broiling

314 Metric Conversion Chart

Liquid Measures Conversion

For foods such as yogurt, applesauce, or cottage cheese, which are not quite liquid but not quite solid, use fluid measures for conversion.

Both systems, the U.S. standard and metric, use spoon measures. The sizes are slightly different, but the difference is not significant in general cooking. (It may, however, be significant in baking.)

tbsp = tablespoon   tsp = teaspoon   c = cup

Spoons, cups, pints, quarts	Fluid ounces (oz)	Milliliters (ml), deciliters (dl), and liters (l); rounded off
1 tsp	⅙	5 ml
3 tsp (1 tbsp)	½	15 ml
1 tbsp	½	¼ dl (or 1 tbsp)
4 tbsp (¼ c)	2	½ dl (or 4 tbsp)
⅓ c	2⅔	¾ dl
½ c	4	1 dl
¾ c	6	1¾ dl
1 c	8	250 ml (or ¼ L)
2 c (1 pint)	16	500 ml (or ½ L)
4 c (1 quart)	32	1 L
4 qt (1 gallon)	128	3¾ L

Solid Measures Conversion

Converting solid measures between U.S. standard and metric is not as straightforward as it might seem. The density of the substance being measured makes a big difference in the volume to weight conversion. For example, 1 tablespoon of flour is ¼ ounce and 8.75 grams, whereas 1 tablespoon of butter or shortening is ½ ounce and 15 grams. The following chart is intended as a guide only. Some experimentation may be necessary to achieve success.

Formulas for conversion:
Ounces to grams: Multiply ounces by 28.35
Grams to ounces: Multiply grams by 0.035

Ounces	Pounds	Grams	Kilograms
1		30	
4	¼	115	
8	½	225	
9		250	¼
12	¾	430	
16	1	450	
18		500	½
	2¼	1000	1
	5		2¼
	10		4½

Linear Measures Conversion

Pan sizes are very different in countries that use metric versus the U.S. standard. This is more significant in baking than in general cooking.

Formulas for conversion:
Inches to centimeters: Multiply inches by 2.54.
Centimeters to inches: Multiply centimeters by 0.39.

Inches	Centimeters	Inches	Centimeters
½	1½	9	23
1	2½	10	25
2	5	12 (1 ft.)	30
3	8	14	35
4	10	15	38½
5	13	16	40
6	15	18	45
7	18	20	50
8	20	24 (2 ft.)	60

Index